Praise for

CONVERGENCE HEALING

"With a gentle touch, Peter Bedard teaches us how to look inside and tap into astounding powers of healing and intuition that we've had within us all along."

—Gerry Katzman, award-winning
comedy teacher and actor

"Compelling and concisely written, *Convergence Healing* speaks directly to the core of the reader's being, allowing not only understanding of one's own pain, be it of mind, body and/or spirit, but allowing the reader to grasp the message that pain carries. The book contains case studies, wherein Peter has successfully worked with individuals in healing their deep-rooted pain through the application of his method. And the exercises in the pages are practical, straightforward, and profound. *Convergence Healing* is a must-read for all who seek to heal their pain [...] with understanding and love instead of hate and fear."

—Steven Maines, author of The Trilogy of the Spear,
a.k.a. The Merlin Factor Trilogy

"Convergence Healing is really helping me get through what has held me back for so long.... I am leaning into the fear, and the pain is subsiding."

—Mary E. Kennedy, host/executive producer
of the *Oh, Mary!* show

"In *Convergence Healing,* Peter Bedard and Brian Sheffield Hunt give anyone who suffers a road map for eliminating the pain by listening to its message in order to heal on every level—physical, mental, emotional, and spiritual. The two main tenants of Convergence Healing are 'changing your thinking about your pain . . . and using this new point of view to propel you into healthy action.' It's a great read."

—Connie Kaplan, author of *The Invisible Garment* and
The Woman's Book of Dreams

"What a wonderful gem of a book! So thoughtfully written and inspiring. The perfect handbook for anyone seeking physical, emotional, and spiritual wellness."

—Kelle James, author of *Smile for the Camera*

"There could not be a more appropriate time for this exceptionally brilliant book to be here to enlighten the world. Bedard has created an eye-opening classic—capturing the true essence of how embracing our HEALTH is about the deprogramming pain process to LET THE HATE HEAL through owning our journey to LOVE—allowing us to EVOLVE."

—Sharita Star, author, astrologer & numerologist

"This book is a must-read for anyone looking to permanently heal on the deepest levels. Peter's natural, proven, and powerful method of healing will help many. This simple yet life-altering practice is a fast-track to a healthy, whole, pain-free life that we all deserve."

—Melissa Rebronja, certified life coach & hypnotist

"As a full-time stay-at-home dad, I don't have a lot of time for myself. I had to work through physical and emotional pain but didn't want it to take away from my parenting abilities. What helped me most was the section on 'How to Navigate out of Your Fog,' as it taught actionable steps that were doable and direct, and my life and my family life are better for it."

—Joël Mejia, 3jsand1s.com

"Peter's book gave me a new way to deal with my back pain. I was in a car accident two years ago and thought my life would be filled with pain forever. So I looked up the exercises in the book and practiced them daily. [Convergence Healing] gave me a new lease on life and a more evolved way to deal with my recovery."

—Jason Stuart, actor & comedian

"Peter Bedard's new book, *Convergence Healing,* is powerful and life changing! I highly recommend this book for anyone interested in healing pain from their mind and body."

—Gary Quinn, life coach, television producer, and bestselling author of *The YES Frequency* and *May the Angels Be with You*

"*Convergence Healing* is an extraordinary book that can help heal your pain, heal your thoughts, and improve your life."

—Tim Braun, international medium and
author of *Life and Death*

"Convergence Healing allows one to see and understand how our pain can serve us in the most powerful and healing ways. This book is a road map and guide to help people live their best and most-fulfilling lives. It is beautifully written, and provides the reader with such incredible hope. It is a must-read for anyone who wants to heal emotionally, mentally, physically, and spiritually."

—Erica Spiegelman, author of *Rewired*

"The convergence of mind, body, and spirit could not be made more seamless and digestible. Thank you, Peter, for a delightful journey into the light of wholeness and health. We would expect no less from one of our star graduates."

—George Kappas, M.A., M.F.T.,
Director/HMI College of Hypnotherapy

"Convergence Healing has given me a whole new way of looking at and dealing with issues that I have fought with unsuccessfully for years. Peter's techniques are truly breakthroughs, very powerful and life changing. Everybody needs Convergence Healing."

—Patti Negri, author, psychic, medium, and producer

"Peter Bedard's passion and commitment to helping others is on display in *Convergence Healing*. In [Peter's] telling his own story with honesty and pairing it with case studies, the reader is given a vision of recovery from one's past pain. The quality of his work is evident in the exercises: uncomplicated and applicable. It is awesome to witness his insights into humanity, and I recommend this book to anyone looking to move forward in their life."
—Scott Sandland, HypnoThoughts.com

"Peter's grasp of a variety of different cultures and scientifically valid approaches make it possible [for readers] to navigate through some of the toughest times in life, and embrace them not only as a learning experience but as a journey and a necessity. As a doctor who has been responsible for some of the most powerful celebrities and international dignitaries in the world, I recognize and clinically utilize what [Peter] discusses in regard to not only forgiving the 'enemy' of your story, but also forgiving oneself for the choices made leading up to that story. Exceptional work, and a digestible and usable read. Well done, Peter."
—Dr. Grace H. Hameister, DC

"In an age of over medication, instantaneous stress, and thin solutions, it is both enlightening and empowering to have *Convergence Healing* at your disposal. Peter Bedard is a gem of a human and this book is a genuine extension of his knowledge, soul, experience, and expertise!"
—Kevin E. West, founder of the Actors' Network

CONVERGENCE HEALING

HEALING PAIN WITH ENERGETIC LOVE

Peter Bedard, M.A., C.Ht.
WITH Brian Sheffield Hunt

Foreword by Dr. Mary Helen Hensley

ENLIVEN BOOKS
—
ATRIA
New York   London   Toronto   Sydney   New Delhi

ENLIVEN

An Imprint of Simon & Schuster, Inc.
1230 Avenue of the Americas
New York, NY 10020

First Enliven Books trade paperback edition December 2015

ENLIVEN BOOKS and colophon are trademarks of Simon & Schuster, Inc.

For information about special discounts for bulk purchases,
please contact Simon & Schuster Special Sales at 1-866-506-1949
or business@simonandschuster.com.

The Simon & Schuster Speakers Bureau can bring authors to your live event. For
more information or to book an event, contact the Simon & Schuster Speakers
Bureau at 1-866-248-3049 or visit our website at www.simonspeakers.com.

Interior design by Kyoko Watanabe

Manufactured in the United States of America

10   9   8   7   6   5   4   3   2   1

Library of Congress Cataloging-in-Publication Data

Names: Bedard, Peter Albert.
Title: Convergence healing : healing pain with energetic love / Peter Bedard
   with Brian Sheffield Hunt ; foreword by Mary Helen Hensley.
Description: First Edition. | New York : Atria/Enliven Books, 2015.
Subjects: LCSH: Pain. | Energy medicine. | Healing. | BISAC: HEALTH & FITNESS
   / Alternative Therapies. | HEALTH & FITNESS / Pain Management. | BODY,
   MIND & SPIRIT / Healing / General.
Classification: LCC BF515 .B394 2015 | DDC 615.8/52—dc23 LC record available
   at http://lccn.loc.gov/2015039507

ISBN 978-1-5011-1952-1
ISBN 978-1-5011-1953-8 (ebook)

To my parents,
and to everyone who perseveres through their pain with love
and
to the pain itself for giving me such a blessed life

Find a place inside where there's joy and
the joy will burn out the pain.

—JOSEPH CAMPBELL

CONTENTS

CONTENTS

FOREWORD

In the autumn of 2013, I had the privilege of being asked to speak at the Cure What Ails You conference aboard the majestic *Queen Mary*, in Long Beach, California. The other speakers, all at the top of their respective fields, were presenting their cutting-edge methods for healing physical, emotional, and spiritual pain. One after another, these healers captivated the audience with their vitality and enthusiasm and, especially, with the riveting case studies they shared about people who had finally liberated themselves from lives defined by crushing pain and who began to live, instead, with authentic vitality and joy.

Just as I was finishing my own presentation and moving toward the back of the hall, my attention turned to a speaker who was talking about his death experience. I was stopped in my tracks. The speaker was Peter Bedard, and his own experience was so hauntingly similar to my own that I realized I was in the presence of a true kindred spirit. Peter is beautiful, charismatic, and passionate, and I felt compelled to turn back and move toward him as he talked about how nearly dying for good propelled him into a state of such all-encompassing pain that he nearly lost himself in his own terrible suffering.

Peter was utterly honest in sharing how he had allowed himself to become a victim to his pain, how the terrible vehicular crash he was in not only broke up his body, which nearly cost him his life, but led him into a very dangerous mind-set that distorted his thinking in ways that dominated his life for the next several decades. I listened intently as he described his pain, fear, and anger and recounted what a destructive force blame had become on his reality. I found myself nodding in recognition, as I, too, at one point had been a committed victim, blaming things outside myself for the disappointments I experienced in my life.

Peter began to talk about how healing is an inside job, and how each of us must wake up to the fact that we, and we alone, are responsible for healing what ails us. Then he outlined the step-by-step method he'd used to retrain his own mind and shared that, by taking control of his own thought processes, he was able to make positive changes, take more meaningful actions, and create a more fulfilling life. The resulting liberation he experienced has been nothing less than astounding. This was my first introduction to Peter and his revolutionary program of Convergence Healing.

Now I am blessed to call Peter my dear friend, and I'm equally blessed to have had the firsthand experience of implementing his simple yet powerful steps of personal growth and positive change in my own life. I am thrilled that Peter decided to write this book, so that I can share Convergence Healing with my clients and my dearest loved ones.

My deepest gratitude goes out to Peter, as well as Brian Sheffield Hunt, for creating such a tangible, realistic, and actionable set of tools that I can recommend with the greatest confidence. I am certain that this book will be the catalyst for change in many lives, starting with your own. Let the healing begin!

—*Dr. Mary Helen Hensley*
Athlone, Ireland

My Convergence Healing

When Peter brought me on as his coauthor, I knew very little about his work. I figured that I would spend some time with a bright fellow, brush up on a few good life skills, turn in the book's manuscript promptly, and be on my way to the next new and interesting job. Instead, I now literally organize my life into "before *Convergence Healing*" and "after *Convergence Healing*."

You see, instead of partnering on this self-help book with a writer who already had his own hearty grasp on his mental, physical, and spiritual well-being, Peter took the more challenging route; he would be working alongside a writer who was bogged down by unique, finely aged insecurities and plagued with anxiety issues that ran so deep they often left me unable to write for hours or days at a time. What could possibly go wrong?

Somehow, I had learned to live with a nearly crippling brew of unresolved trauma that felt like it was an integral part of myself. When I began working with Peter, my concept of who I was began to sort itself out; this is sometimes the unexpected bonus of working with a gifted expert. As I got to know Peter and his healing methodology, my mind began to open up and unfold like a flower. I felt like I was on the verge of some huge shift, but of course change didn't initially look the way I hoped it would.

Early in my work with Peter, a long-term business partnership of mine began to crumble just as the project that I had poured my heart and soul into was about to really launch. I tried everything I could think of to salvage the situation, but eventually all my efforts (and the project) led nowhere. This was devastating for me professionally, but it also fed the insecure child trapped inside of me, the little boy who had been bullied and teased and who always feared and prepared for the worst.

I realized that this was the true gift of working alongside Peter; finally I would learn how to mend my broken spirit and restore my untrusting heart.

Peter and I began to meet every Wednesday morning in a beautiful shaded park. I felt so lucky sitting across a stone picnic table from a perfectly flawed human being who had done the hard work of learning how to get out of his own way. He let his pain guide him to a way of being in the world that was truly joyful and free. Through Peter's example, I began to understand that if I was willing to not only pay attention to my pain but do so in a more loving way, instead of automatically drugging it or scorning it, my pain could tell me what it needed to heal.

Peter believes in integration. He believes in calling all the lost, disparate, rejected pieces of ourselves home. He believes that we can and should feel "as one" in our own bodies. As I began to personally experience what he was talking about, I agreed with and began to trust Peter and his process more and more. We came to call his method Convergence Healing.

I was no easy convert. In fact, I came to my work with Peter full of skepticism. There he was, Peter Bedard, hypnotherapist extraordinaire, sitting across from me, outlining his method of healing and telling me how gratifying it has been for him to watch thousands of people benefit from it. Meanwhile, there I was, smiling and nodding my head while a chorus of traitorous voices flooded my thoughts with doubt and disbelief.

The harder Peter and I worked together, the more my subconscious tried to stave off change of any kind, healthy or not. Convergence Healing was going to work very nicely for Peter's clients—it just would not work for me. The resistance I faced was formidable.

Even though I was racked with pain and paranoia, had recently lost the hair at my crown and was sporting a new bald spot, and was having trouble sleeping for the first time in my life, my subconscious wanted nothing to do with change. Sure, my "comfort zone" was suffocating me, but I was a good prisoner and had no intention of leaving the oppressive emotional prison that my pain had constructed around me.

But then, some really transformative shifts began to happen.

One of the bedrock tenets of Peter's process is that each of us wields power that we must learn to harness and use for our higher good, mentally, physically, and spiritually. I had to take responsibility and acknowledge how powerful my thoughts were. I had to commit to better, wiser thinking and give up being a languid slave to automatic negative thoughts.

Initially, I was afraid to accept this potent call to action. Once I picked up that one of the first keys to creating my own health was becoming more mindful of my everyday thinking, little but no less miraculous things started to happen: my finances flourished, highly regarded people stepped forward to support my creative work, and someone even offered me a beautiful, serene space in which to work. By assuming personal responsibility for my thinking, I was beginning to care for my overall well-being. I had taken my first step.

Convergence Healing entails giving up any identity as "the victim" in our own lives. To do this, I needed to identify the habitual dysfunctional behavioral loops that kept me from getting beyond the cycle of feeling wounded, which always led to me feeling worse than before. By providing actionable lessons and tools to help strip away any need for blame, I was able to let go of the "poor me" Brian I had become so fond of. This was radically freeing.

The more Peter taught me about the way the subconscious mind actually operates, the more I was able to identify all of the really ingenious distractions I had created so that I would not have to recognize the pain I was in. Suddenly, I was onto myself. I was beginning to get that it did not matter what self-sabotaging behavior I engaged in. Whatever it was, it only served to keep the focus off myself. Just like the rest of the human race, I had created a nearly limitless array of "beards" that cloaked my true pain from me and kept me from getting the message my pain so desperately needed me to understand. Unfortunately, these crafty techniques only pull us further away from our true selves and seriously hamper any ability to live the lives of dignity and grace we all yearn for.

Next, I had to get comfortable with all my discomfort, and there was a lot of it. Once I made the commitment, however, I got curious and found that I was talking to myself in the car a lot. I dialogued with my gnarly, unhappy parts and learned to understand and make peace with them. Sure, I got a few weird looks in traffic, but for once, I did not care about what others were thinking of me. I was too energized dismantling my old ways of thinking.

In one mind-blowing mini-conversation, I took a moment to

assure the knee of my slightly shorter leg, the knee that always gave me problems, that I loved and appreciated it as much as the knee on my slightly longer (stronger) leg. Instantly, and I mean instantly, I felt a rush of energy surge into my knee—it felt tingly, warm, and *right*, like it was filling in an empty space that had needed filling for a long time. I have never had any problems with my knee since.

With my sense of responsibility in regard to my health clearly in the right space, with no whiny sense of victimhood allowed (for very long)—and armed with the knowledge that my pain is something that must be listened to and honored so it can finally heal—I was able to carefully craft my intention for perfect health. For me, this last step became a very important reminder, a beacon in the dark to rely upon whenever I felt sad, lazy, or sentimental for the blissfully ignorant sod I used to be.

As I mentioned earlier, the universe seemed more than willing to support my new, healthier goals. It was like the net would not appear unless I made the firm decision to take my health into my own hands and really go for it. I was so sick of living half a life and never believing that anything wonderful was meant for me.

At times, I was furious and restless. Other times, I was sad and lethargic. The more Peter's first steps resonated within me, the more I began to notice that I was beginning to act, feel, and behave better.

I like to use the image of a gum ball machine to illustrate my own transformation. Before I met Peter, my gum ball machine was filled with the black, stale memories and imprints of my previous experiences. Every morning, these would drop into my mind and fill my head with terrible thoughts, sometimes before my feet even hit the floor. Several months into my healing process, the gum ball machine began to fill with a fresh rainbow assortment of thoughts and feelings. Oh, there were still some black gum balls in the mix, but they were not the only thoughts that would drop out of my subconscious upon waking.

Every morning after I shower, I clean the water spots off the glass shower door with a squeegee. I loathe this task, but I get into trouble if I do not do it. Once I had committed to the Convergence Healing path, I realized I could dedicate this time to a mini-meditation and verbally express how happy, healthy, and grateful I felt for my life, all while performing a daily chore that I usually hate.

I stopped listening to depressing news on the radio and stuck to classical music. I found that my time in the garden could do so much more for my spirit than I ever realized if I stayed more present while being there. While my senses felt heightened in a curious way, I also felt more connected to everything around me.

Here I was, making little changes and adjustments to my thinking while performing many of the same tasks I had always done, but now, all those little moments seemed more real and meaningful to me. I began to go through days where I did not even know how to feel or act outside of the overbearing, shrill, negative voice in my head reminding me that everyone knows that I suck. Instead, Peter kept encouraging me to take control of my mind and use my thoughts to support a new, healthier way of living.

I felt more alive with everything I was doing, from writing to brushing my teeth to gardening to washing dishes. It was like everything mattered more because I was actively bonding with everything around me instead of being so afraid. I know that sounds corny, but it is very true. (It is no coincidence that my garden also looked more fabulous than ever.) My vibrant flowers are, to me, an accurate reflection of all my positive interior changes.

My energy level felt like it came from a deeper, much more potent source, like it was no longer just me pouring fuel into my tank. I was somehow receiving help from a power higher than me, Peter, or his program. I felt connected. The more hang-ups I let go of, the faster I responded to banishing bad thoughts, and the less pain I was in. I was flabbergasted at how long the list was of things that no longer bothered me so much, which Peter had asked me to put together.

Now that I was calmer and more centered, it was time to incorporate the final steps of Peter's compassionate healing program into my daily regimen. I still had to develop mind, body, and spirit exercises for myself. God bless the universe, for it really seemed to be reaching out to support me.

On the mind level, I had been examining my thinking for a while by working with a talented psychotherapist. I did not let up on this, and my work got deeper, messier, and more real and intense. With him, I was learning to appreciate and like myself again, in spite of my faults.

At a party I almost did not go to, I met a teacher who leads healing meditation sessions, just two blocks from my home. So I went. Meditation, something I had never before taken seriously, really clears the mind and helps me hear myself better. Some days, after meditating, I feel as if my mind has been massaged. I am definitely more comfortable with silence. My discernment is keener. I can sense when a thought or a behavior is not going to enhance my health, and so I'm able to redirect myself before I take that misstep.

As for my body exercises, one day I discovered a newly renovated park with exercise equipment and a track only four blocks away from my house. And just driving by it, I found that my body craved exercise.

So I began jogging. Jogging in the morning lets my body know that I am willing to start each day focused on my health. The repetition of the laps I run helps me work on my patience. Seeing so many dogs at the park makes my soul smile. Mind, body, and spirit are all being addressed as I run my measly ten laps. Wait, I mean as I run my *mighty* ten laps.

On a spirit level, I realized that I wanted to begin reading fiction books for fun again. I had not picked up a book simply because it tickled my fancy in years. I did not realize how much I missed the decadence of dedicating an afternoon to getting lost in a good, old-fashioned story. I also made regular dates with myself to visit used-book stores. There is nothing like them!

More changes for the better kept happening, and I could not deny it. Was all this actually due to engaging in these various Convergence Healing practices? I believe the answer is a resounding yes.

My own Convergence Healing continues to be incredibly life-changing. I feel happy and optimistic (again) and am determined not to get in my own way (anymore). Convergence Healing is easy to follow, totally noninvasive, and deeply soulful. Now, whenever I recognize some kind of pain, be it mental, physical, or more, I pay careful attention. You too will learn that pain is not the enemy and in fact may be your greatest teacher. Thank you, Peter!

—*Brian Sheffield Hunt*

CHAPTER ONE

The Gift of Pain

Pain can only feed on pain. Pain cannot feed on joy. It finds it quite indigestible.

—Eckhart Tolle

Where does it hurt?

I know this seems like an odd way to begin a book, but I honestly want to know: Are you, at this very moment, experiencing some kind of pain? Is your heart aching? Are your bones or back bothering you? Is your spirit agitated or restless? I'm guessing that, more than likely, you are murmuring yes.

That's because pain is the great unifier and leveler; all of us wonderful human beings, no matter how rich, smart, or loved we are, experience debilitating pain at some point in our lives. This pain may be physical, or it may be spiritual or emotional. Or it may be all three. What I've come to understand is that pain is one of the most potent forces we will ever encounter, and I've devoted my life to helping as many people as I can understand that pain can be a force for good.

So, tell me. Are you in pain?

When I recently posed the question to a circle of friends, the range of responses I received confirmed what I've come to know: all of us experience pain in one form or another, and most of us allow our pain to limit our beliefs about who we are and what we can do. Here are a smattering of the responses I received:

> "The first thing that comes to my mind is limitation. Not being able to do what I want because of being in too much physical pain."
>
> "I knew I was in intense pain when I did not feel anything. I could tell it was my body protecting me from something it knew I could not handle yet."
>
> "The first thing that comes to mind when I think of pain is the horrible pain of addiction—right before I finally waved the white flag. No physical pain has ever come close."
>
> "Root canal!!!!!!"
>
> "The pain of losing a loved one. For me, it was almost unbearable."
>
> "When I think of pain, I think of being alone. That is the worst possible pain."

According to data released by the International Association for the Study of Pain and the European Pain Federation and endorsed by the World Health Organization, pain reportedly affects one in five people worldwide in the form of mostly moderate to severe chronic pain. With one-fifth of the globe's population suffering, it is no wonder that we are forever on the hunt for newer and better ways to secure relief from our pain.

Over two thousand years ago, the early Greeks and Romans were developing rudimentary ideas about the role our brain plays in producing the perception of pain and ways to counteract this influence. In the nineteenth century, opiates such as morphine were widely used to relieve pain, and German chemist Felix Hoffmann developed the first medically useful form of aspirin from a substance in willow bark. Today, aspirin remains the most commonly used pain reliever and is, in and of itself, a billion-dollar global drug business. And then, of course, there are the opioids such as Oxycontin, which remain overly prescribed despite the high risk of addiction. During my own struggle with chronic pain, I was offered but refused many drugs. It wasn't until I went in and made peace with the person I was while in pain that I was able to find relief from my pain—without ever needing to pick up a substance, get surgery, or in any other way alter my mind or body.

Convergence Healing is about learning to listen to the wisdom your pain has to share, and allowing this wisdom to unlock those parts of yourself that have been shut down, hidden, or otherwise disenfranchised so that you can heal and become whole again.

Pain is the ultimate paradox. When we injure ourselves, we feel broken. And we are broken at those moments, but usually not in the ways that we think. That is because pain can be misleading, distracting, or downright deceiving if we don't meet it head-on. What you will learn in *Convergence Healing* is how to face your pain's power with your own personal power. When you do this, you will realize that you are more than your pain.

What exactly is pain? Is it a cluster of nerve endings that have been traumatized? Is it an unmet need or longing in our hearts? Is it an unhelpful yet deeply entrenched train of thought? A basic, clinical definition describes pain as "the physical feeling caused by disease, injury, or something that hurts the body." A secondary definition goes a bit further, adding that pain can also be "sadness caused by mental or emotional suffering."

The Latin word *poena*, the origin for our English word "pain," means penalty or suffering inflicted as punishment for an offense. In Greek mythology, Poine was a lesser goddess of retribution, vengeance, and punishment. Many ancient cultures believed pain and disease were punishment for human folly. To rid people of pain, ancient healers used magic and spiritualism in an attempt to appease angry gods, often by engaging in rituals, offerings, and sacrifices that involved a lot of pain. In ancient times, the thinking went: What are you willing to suffer and sacrifice to be rid of your pain?

Today, we think of pain as a symptom that should be eliminated as quickly as possible. We spend a lot of time thinking about how to avoid or not feel our pain. So we turn to drugs, surgery, and a whole host of unhealthy behaviors (drinking, overeating, overspending), believing that if we can just wipe out whatever pain we are feeling, we will be good to go.

Unfortunately, we have it all wrong. Yes, pain is a symptom of something larger that ails us. It is absolutely a messenger of sorts. How will we ever get the message if we shoot (or medicate) the messenger before we have given it a chance to speak? In other words, in our modern world, which favors numbing out over raw, real experience, we are too eager to eliminate pain and so we miss out on gleaning the wisdom it has for us. Paradoxically, when we focus on suppressing our pain without knowing what it really is, we make it all the stronger. This is when physical pain or mental anguish (negative thinking) overwhelm us and become chronic. This is when we lose ourselves to pain.

All of us experience pain. It is a fundamental experience of being a living, breathing person on this planet. There are basically two types of pain we may experience. Acute pain is short, sharp, and often very shocking. This is the kind of pain we experience when we are in a car accident or when we are struck by an intense medical condition, such as appendicitis. Acute pain is usually associated with physical injury, like the excruciating pain of breaking a bone or the crushing experience of having a car door slammed on your finger. Cells in the injured tissue at the site of impact emit chemicals that activate local nerve endings. The stirred-up nerve endings send an electrochemical impulse via the nerves to the spinal cord. The impulse then travels to the thalamus part of the brain and continues on to its destination, the cerebral cortex. This type of pain is relatively straightforward—and short-lived. It is a complex set of neurological reactions that give us a very clear message. Ouch! Stop what you are doing and pay attention to me!

Chronic pain is the more insidious kind of pain because it tends to outwit and outlast whatever Western treatments we throw at it. Typically starting out as a physical reaction to some form of accident or trauma, chronic pain, whatever its origin, tends to latch onto our psyches with a vengeance, taking us hostage. Our pain, if left untreated and allowed to become chronic, can take us over—body, mind, and soul. If we are not careful, it can actually become us.

We humans tend to experience pain in the three most important realms of our existence: the physical, the emotional, and the spiritual. Sometimes pain that begins in one realm bleeds into another and we experience pain on several levels at once. For example, a woman who was abused suffers deep emotional and psychic pain, but she may also experience physical pain in her lower back or pelvic floor. A man who was unable to protect his family from physical harm may suffer from seemingly unrelated severe neck and shoulder pain, which masks the true source of his pain—his core emotional trauma. Or, an athlete who strains her knee may feel the emotional anguish of having let her teammates down when she is unable to compete with them. Inevitably, when one part of us is injured, it has a domino effect on the other essential parts of ourselves. This is why I believe, from years of working with thousands of clients, that when we experience pain it not only exists on all levels but must be treated on all levels.

Physical pain is the easiest type of pain to identify—and to heal, especially when it involves a superficial wound, one that can be seen by the naked eye. Physical pain, because of its obviousness, is also the type of pain we are less inclined to judge. It is a different story when it comes to emotional or spiritual pain.

Emotional pain is an affective response to a life event. We all understand the pain of grieving, especially when someone loved dies too soon or leaves this planet suddenly. Emotional pain, unlike physical pain, triggers a process that usually needs more time and attention. How many of us have experienced the pain of stubbing a toe as being "no big deal" when compared to the pain we feel when we have been dumped by someone we thought was "the one"? Though no flesh has been torn or blood shed, our hearts are wounded in ways that will inhibit our ability to lead full and fulfilling lives if we do not adequately process that pain.

The same is true of pain that hits us hard on the spiritual level, and this type of pain is, I believe, the most difficult to identify and heal (at least, when using traditional Western methodologies, such as counseling).

In *La Cultura: Conceptual Strategies to Understand Identity, Diversity, Otherness and the Difference*, Patricio Guerrero Arias refers to spiritual pain as the "disruption in the principle which pervades a person's entire being and which integrates and transcends one's biological and psychosocial nature." Christian hospice chaplain Tom Allain's years of experience led him to define spiritual pain as occurring when "there is an event that violates the core values, beliefs, or needs of the person." NANDA International describes spiritual pain as "a state of disorder in a person's inner core. It might be a chronic or an acute heartache, an existential dissonance that expresses itself in behavioral incongruities. An important characteristic is that it is a pain appropriate medication does not relieve." They list the experiential features of spiritual pain as follows:

- Disconnection from others; unwillingness to engage
- Preoccupation with self
- Feeling outcast and alone
- Expressing a loss of future
- Feeling abandoned
- Distress, despair, withdrawal
- No joy in anything
- Pain is fixed
- Feeling trapped
- Anger, shame, guilt

Addressing emotional or spiritual pain is where modern medicine, too, fails us. For example, a young man suffering from sexual dysfunction (physical pain) often has a deep fear of intimacy (emotional pain) and his heart (spiritual pain) feels alone and unloved in the world. A new mother may be hurting from a lack of support from her husband (emotional pain) and as a result be unable to relax and breast-feed her child (physical pain), which may lead her into a deep, postpartum depression (spiritual pain).

In the end, it does not matter where our pain originates. What matters is how we honor our experience of pain and how we listen to what it is trying to teach us. I know this because I let my own pain, a pain that was initially physical but became spiritual and emotional, hold me hostage for most of my life. Until I freed myself with Convergence Healing.

THE NIGHT I DIED

I gaze down at my lifeless body. I am dead. No pulse, no heartbeat, no breath. I am simply dead. I never see this coming. Everything happens so fast.

Tops, I'm traveling twenty miles per hour. I'm riding along a twisty suburban road on my little yellow Motobecane, under the light of a full moon. I am too busy being angry and put out to appreciate the beautiful nighttime scene I am a part of. Lost in my thoughts, I am having a heated, internal argument with my parents. I'm only seventeen years old, but I resent my parents for not trusting me more. I want to go to a cast party, but my parents told me I could not go, so instead I am being the good son and going home.

As I am riding along, fuming, a big car roars up behind me. I lean into a curve in the road ahead as the car's white headlights flash brightly in my side-view mirrors. The light is blinding.

Up ahead, I see too late that a parked semitruck is entirely blocking my way. I am driving near the curb and only a few feet from the rear of the truck when my scooter is bumped from behind. Time strangely slows down as I jump out of my body just before impact and watch the accident unfold in front of me. My body is slammed into the steel tailgate of the semitruck. I float above the side of the road and watch in slow motion as my body smashes into the truck. I watch myself bounce off the rear of the semi and into the middle of the road. There is a strange silence and a profound peace. I notice that my body is not moving.

My scooter, my prized possession, is a mangled yellow metal mess. Blood oozes from my scraped-up face and my knee is bent at a grotesque angle. A budding dancer with my heart set on a Broadway career, I remember thinking, "This cannot be good," though with every second that passes I am more and more detached from any sensation of pain or even an opinion about what is happening in front of me. In fact, I watch these things, feeling a strange deepening sense of peace and calm. I am detached. I am aware that there is pain, but I do not feel any of it.

No one else is on the road. I feel utterly alone yet utterly at peace. I find myself drifting upward and hovering high over the accident. The car that hit me drives off as the stillness of the night returns.

Then I depart.

One second I am calmly awaiting the moment a car runs over and crushes my dead body, the next I am rushing, floating fast along a white otherworldly tunnel. Being drawn down this spinning tunnel of white clouds is absolute bliss. The tunnel corkscrew spins and I am shooting like a comet through it, experiencing love and joy like I have never known. As I ascend through this tunnel of light, I become less and less interested in what I am leaving behind. I am not just at peace. I *am* peace.

I arrive. I am here . . . wherever "here" is. Heaven, or whatever this place is, looks exactly how other people generally describe it. There are no billowy clouds, just massive whiteness. It is soft, brilliantly white, yet diffused. I sense that there is a floor, and that I am standing on it, but I cannot see it. Ceilings and walls do not exist here; there is only brilliance, an inherent living light. I even feel like I am in a defined space . . . if you can somehow define a room made up of infinity. With each passing second my heart beats with more expansive joy.

I begin to explore this place of vast nothingness. I am so curious. My curiosity is overwhelming. . . . It is even fun and it feels like play to explore and try to understand this place. It feels like a lot of time goes by. I feel as though I have been floating in this place of stillness for quite a while.

I start to ask myself where everyone is (I was expecting to see some dead relatives or at least my departed dog), and at that very moment in which I wonder if anyone knows I am here, I see an old man with a long, stringy white beard. He seems to be waiting for me to notice him.

I sense an unfamiliar familiarity about him. I feel as though I know this stranger. No, I do not just know him, I love him. I love him so much, I feel as if my heart is erupting from my chest. This love goes beyond any love I have ever experienced before. It is painful and joyous at the same time. It is felt in every cell of my being.

In this moment I am swept up in the enormity of this love, and it is as if I am meeting God . . . but I know this old man is not God. He is *of* God. He is there to speak with me, but he is not God. He wears a brown tweed suit that is cut like the fashion just before the turn of the nineteenth century. The name Hong Kong pops into my mind. When I am older I come to think of him as Lao-tzu, a dear friend and a wise old man. In this moment he is like an angel, but he is not that either. I understand now that he is a "guide" or even a "guardian." I feel like he is my version of a fairy godmother.

"I know you, right?" I think I am speaking out loud. Or at least it seems like I am—I am not sure. He is translucent, like the holograph of Obi-Wan Kenobi in *Star Wars*, and he has shape and form but he is pure light. Like Princess Leia, I sense this man is "my only hope."

Although I feel deeply connected to this man, I desperately want to see some of my loved ones. I find myself thinking about my great-grandmother who died a month before I was born. Is she here? But I see no one but Lao-tzu in this place of exquisite nothingness.

I know that the fuzzy man with the stringy beard loves me. I feel love in his eyes as he calmly speaks to me. "You have to go back. You are not supposed to be here." For a second, I am confused. Then I am furious. The overwhelming love I have been feeling is replaced in seconds by a deep churning anger.

Back on earth, I do not fit in at church. I do not fit in at home. I definitely do not fit in at school. The only place I have been free to be myself is onstage. And here. And now I am being told I have to leave?

"Fuck you," I say to the bearded man. And then I am gone.

It took decades for me to recognize that the man I had encountered at the end of the white tunnel did not have an agenda; he was simply a messenger. He was not rejecting me because I did not belong. He was letting me know that it just was not my time. Still, I was ready to depart this earth then and I am today. Although I engage in this life as fully as possible, if God, or Lao-tzu, tapped me on the shoulder tomorrow and nodded, saying, "It is time, buddy," I would ask to say a few quick good-byes and then be on my way.

I would love to tell you that my life after my death experience became easier, but in fact the opposite happened. For too many years after I totaled my scooter and nearly died for good, my life mirrored the story of Sisyphus, who cheated the gods and was condemned to roll a boulder uphill every day only to find it at the bottom of the hill the following morning. Ever since I had the experience in the white tunnel, I have also had an ache to get back there, to go back "home." Because of this longing, I wrongly punished myself for everything, including being alive.

I awoke in my body and told the paramedic who was leaning over me, his ear close to my chest, that there was an insurance card in my back pocket and to take me to the hospital. He jumped and let out a yelp when I opened my eyes. I must have scared the crap out of him because he looked panicked, like his eyes were about to pop out of his head.

And then I am gone again, floating above and watching the paramedics load my broken-up body into the ambulance. I watch them close the doors and drive off. With every fiber of my being, I do not want to go with them.

With no intention of following the ambulance to the hospital, I remain hovering over the street, thinking to myself, "I do not want to go back!" I am practically screaming it at the top of my lungs, but there is no one around to hear me. I stay as long as I can.

The next thing I knew, I opened my eyes and found myself staring up at a cheap white dropped ceiling. Mom and Dad were there. We were in a hospital, and I was terrified and ashamed because I felt like I should have been able to do something to avoid all this. I was not good enough, and my accident must have been punishment for something I did wrong. I felt scared and ashamed because I did not want to live. . . .

As I lay in that dreary hospital room racked with terrible physical pain, the doctors informed me that I had shattered a knee and split my wrist. It was not until my knee was healed enough for me to begin the painful physical therapy I needed to learn to walk again that they discovered I had also fractured five vertebrae in my spine.

The initial surgery I had to have on my knee was delayed a week because all the torn and dead skin around it had to heal up before a surgeon could cut through it again (at least, that is what the doctors told me). The hospital used my surgery as a teaching session, and surgeons from across the country flew in to witness my knee being pieced back together like a jigsaw puzzle.

I found that I was crying myself to sleep every night that week and many nights thereafter. I began living and breathing fear. I never let on how miserable I was, because if I did, what was I going to do? Apparently, dying was not an option anymore, especially now that doctors surrounded me. I was terrified of ending up in a wheelchair and never being able to dance again. A full year after the accident, I was still angry at and arguing with God. Not really arguing . . . more like screaming at God. I was, quite simply, in an awful place.

In my mind, I would return to that infinite white space and rage at the bearded man who had turned me away. I had pleaded with my angels about how I did not want to be on this plane anymore. I felt rejected—rejected by love and the greatest sense of peace I had ever experienced—and tossed back into a body full of pain. This was not my idea of a blessed life. All I had now was a broken body, bitterness, and dashed dreams. I had so much anger, and I did not know what to do with it. Over the ensuing years, I would shove down that anger over and over again only to have it come out sideways as more sickness and pain.

Instead of getting "better," my suffering intensified. Hiding in pain, I cut myself off from any real solutions for healing. Actually, it was not that I cut myself off from the right solutions; I simply did not know what they were. All that was offered to me were drugs and surgery. I saw that pain medications were only a temporary fix and that masking the pain only made what really ailed me worse, so I simply did not take any. I just learned to live with the pain. Even after my knee had healed, I felt so bad for so long. My list of sufferings included chronic allergies, arthritis, asthma, chronic pain, depression, anxiety, sciatica, fibromyalgia, a hernia, brain damage, as well as several other life-threatening experiences in which I came close to dying once again.

I had grown up in a working-class household where aspirin and prescription medications were turned to whenever any kind of pain was present. My father, a mailman, had such terrible chronic back pain that Mom always made sure the large-size bottles of pain relievers were in the house. After all, purchasing large quantities is almost always the most economical route to go. Where emotional pain was concerned, my family followed the Catholic tradition of denying pain—of becoming a martyr to pain—rather than turning to face and embrace it. This made growing up as a gay son in a semiconservative religious household very challenging. And very lonely. I always felt like an outsider, like I never fit in or belonged. That is, until I found dance, my calling. I was on my way home from my first professional performance when my leg was shattered.

The best my conscious mind could do with all this information, especially when it was coupled with the fact that I had been kicked out of "heaven" by the bearded messenger, was to decide that I was, somehow, born "wrong." This belief became my greatest source of pain, my internal prison. It would take me years and years before I would be led to the holistic and cutting-edge Western healing modalities that would actually help cure me.

Until that time, I stayed huddled up in a dark, unenlightened space. I clung hard to negative opinions, assumptions, and judgments about others and myself in a futile attempt to guard myself from pain. Essentially, I de-evolved and became a child again, stuck in a frozen and surreal state of survival mode. I punished myself with shame, embarrassment, and the overwhelmingly painful belief that I was not good enough.

Years later, once I finally began to understand that true healing is something that we all must take ownership of for ourselves, I trusted myself enough to ignore the advice of the doctors who were too quick to take out the prescription pad and too eager to schedule the next surgery to "clean up" my arthritic, inflamed knee. Instead, I finally turned within and decided to trust that voice inside me that said "There is a better way," even though I had no firm grasp on what that way would be.

No matter where I turned, I bumped into pain. Finally, I hit such a severe low point that I understood I had become a complete victim to pain. I knew that I had no choice but to discover a better way of living.

Now I can see that pain was calling me to heal and love myself. The pain was trying to get my attention, enlighten me, and teach me a deep lesson. Perhaps even my life lesson. My pain actually wanted to set me free. Only I could unlatch the gate to my inner prison, a prison I had unwittingly built myself.

I took a leap of faith that miserable day. In my mind, someday I would find whatever it was that I specifically needed to feel better. Not heal one hundred percent, just feel a bit better for a little while. Gradually, the stronger I got and the better I felt, I understood that I was meant to embrace every part of my being with full, radical acceptance. That it was my job to integrate the lonely, isolated, and wounded parts of myself and make them whole. Only then would the pain that had had me so pinned down dissolve and leave.

Now I refuse to settle. If ever I feel sick, I do not settle for anything less than total wellness. It may take time to restore that sense of wholesome wellness, but because I am so committed to living in the present, I realize I have all the time in the world. It is a new and wonderfully strange experience to live in the moment and feel truly at peace with how things are while still holding a vision of what it will one day feel like to be completely restored, happy, healthy, and free.

Once I made the commitment to take control of my thinking, I was able to see that not only was I living with pain but I was also living in the fear of being in pain for the rest of my life. What a self-defeating load of crap. Somehow, I had become completely maladjusted, a true victim's victim, and I finally saw how suffocating and toxic my belief systems had become.

In the infancy of my rising awareness, whenever negative thoughts presented themselves and threatened to overpower my thinking/behavior/day, I reminded myself to let go of the fear. "Faith, not fear" became my mantra. It sure as hell was better than whatever I had used as a mantra before. I started to believe that my life could be restored and that I could and would find love. Maybe not the love I had experienced when I died, but a love that is alive deep inside of me. Now I wake up every day and strive to experience that love. I find it in the deepest parts of me and usually most passionately when I decide to embrace the most flawed and ugly parts of who I am.

As I began to take charge and turn my health around, I experienced a lot of unexpected guilt. Choosing my own path felt like turning my back on the entrenched doctrines I had been raised with.

Was I betraying my parents somehow? Did the doctors really know better than I did? In spite of all this, I resolved to remain true to my new belief that there had to be more I could do to help myself heal.

What I finally came to understand is that pain is not just a fact of life; it is a gateway to life. We need to approach our own pain with loving curiosity and clear-sightedness. Pain is neither good nor bad—it just is. It is a messenger, from the core of our being, telling us that something needs to be healed. It's calling us to take action.

I do not know why, but the human mind does everything possible to avoid pain. The nervous system and even the subconscious mind get involved in hiding our pain from us, and so we get hijacked into looking into the wrong remedies for our pain (or, in fact, we may treat something utterly unrelated—the symptom—to our deepest pain). Finally, though, researchers, doctors, and therapists are finding more and more that physical pain, even what is called "bony" pain, can and often does originate in a place that has seemingly nothing to do with the area that is feeling the pain.

Noted Washington State back surgeon Dr. David S. Hanscom is canceling or postponing surgeries and asking his clients to try healing themselves with his "Prehab" system, which focuses on sleep, stress management, and cognitive behavioral therapy work.

The famous Dr. Wayne Dyer commonly recommended diet and exercise before turning to prescription drugs.

Buddhist teacher Pema Chödrön encourages us to "lean into our pain." She says: "Feelings like disappointment, embarrassment, irritation, resentment, anger, jealousy, and fear, instead of being bad news, are actually very clear moments that teach us where it is that we're holding back. They teach us to perk up and lean in when we feel we would rather collapse and back away. Painful feelings are like messengers that show us, with terrifying clarity, exactly where we are stuck. This very moment is the perfect teacher, and lucky for us, it is with us wherever we are."

As you move deeper and deeper into Convergence Healing with me, you will be asked to step outside whatever makes up your comfort zone. You will be asked to take an honest inventory of how you think and how you feel and, most important, to identify what is truly causing your pain.

If this sounds daunting, all you have to do is ask yourself the questions I was ultimately forced to ask myself: Do I honestly want to feel better? Do I want to stop being in so much pain? For me, the answer was a plain and truthful yes. It was like a roar permeated my being.

Healing takes work. It requires determination and dedication and the belief that you can do it. Healing is a process, a process of bringing the wounded and hidden parts of yourself out into the light so that they can be freed from shame, guilt, blame, and so many other negative emotions we entrap them in.

Pain will visit you, time and time again, during this precious lifetime. That is what great messengers do. When you understand this, your convergence, your integration, and your healing will begin. It is time.

JACKIE

Sometimes life piles up on you. My client Jackie was experiencing a major pileup. In her late fifties, she found herself lost and miserable. All the things that she used to do in order to avoid pain just did not work anymore.

In her twenties, Jackie had used sex, drugs, and partying to avoid having to face what ailed her. As the years went by, she turned to food, pharmaceutical drugs, and even becoming a workaholic. These tactics all lasted for periods of time but never for long. It was becoming harder and harder to avoid the heavy pain that Jackie was carrying around.

Jackie had been avoiding pain for so long that she was not even sure what she was hiding from anymore. Her life seemed like a blur of shockingly painful events, all stacked up one on top of the other. Her father was distant and unloving. Her mother was an abusive alcoholic. Her brother teased her relentlessly. Her bosses sexually harassed her. Her friends died one after the other in the 1980s due to the AIDS epidemic. Her surviving friends betrayed her trust. The *universe* seemed to be beating Jackie up . . . or was it?

Jackie absorbed each of these experiences, one after the other. She even held on to them, as each trauma felt like a way to be connected to those she had lost. She felt so numb inside that at least the pain reminded her that she was alive.

Yet, at the same time, she would run away from all of these stuffed emotions, too afraid that they would overwhelm her. The thought was that if she gave in and felt the pain, it would become never ending and unbearable. She was in a conundrum; she needed the pain in order to feel at least something and not completely shut down, yet she remained afraid that if she let in any more of the pain, then it would overtake her.

When I asked Jackie how this pain was helping her, she looked at me like I was crazy. From Jackie's perspective, her pain was destroying her life; she couldn't see what I saw, which was that she had become addicted to her pain.

When I met Jackie, she was living with a cancerous tumor. She had been at stage IV for some time and was resigned to living in this "worst-case" state and managing the physical pain she was in.

Even in treating her tumor, Jackie was looking for outside sources to heal her. She started with Western medical doctors (chemo, radiation, surgery) and moved on to psychics and energy healers. When she came to see me, she was deeply involved in a Buddhist prayer group. She had a degree of success with each of these modalities, but, like most everything else in her life, they only went so far. None of them were able to cure Jackie and none of them were able to give her the peace that she claimed to so desire.

When I asked Jackie to look at the pain, her tumor, from a different perspective, she was highly skeptical. How could this thing that was killing her be of benefit and, furthermore, how could she be expected to accept this as a part of her to be loved and respected? After some coaxing, she became willing to try to change her perspective. This is when things really started to happen.

When Jackie approached her pain with respect and curiosity instead of rejection and fear, all kinds of important information began budding toward the surface. As we went through all the injustices and abuse that Jackie had endured in her life, a common thread began to emerge. Beneath all the pain was a simple request from the universe: Jackie needed to love herself unconditionally.

Her pain was no longer something to avoid but actually something to be nurtured. It was a cosmic messenger asking Jackie to heal her wounded heart. Jackie had spent so much time running away from her pain that she never realized it might want to help her resolve some of the issues that had kept her from finding peace in her life.

From this place of new understanding, we began to develop a game plan for how Jackie could acknowledge that she had received and fully comprehended this message. But Jackie had no idea how to be loved. She truly had no idea what love felt like. No wonder she was so comfortable living in that numbed-out space between slouching through life and staving off death.

Our focus quickly shifted from Jackie's cancer to learning what in life gave her the experience of feeling loved. Her pain, brought on by the tumor that was perceived to be killing her, was actually calling out for Jackie to not only survive but also to really live! The tumor gave Jackie the gift of learning to be kind and loving to herself and to spread this sense of happiness instead of lapsing into pity and self-reproach.

Jackie had always wanted to dance, and knowing that at stage IV she might not have much time, her pain prompted her to get on her feet and take those tap dance classes. She'd always wanted to have a dog, but her family frowned upon dogs. The tumor cleared away all the "should nots," and Jackie got a dog.

The more she turned toward her pain with the intention of understanding and honoring it, the more Jackie discovered what it was like to really be alive. Her pain taught her to live in the moment, to appreciate what she had, and to forgive her parents and her brother for not being more loving with her, for not helping her to learn the skill of loving herself. The gift of the tumor and the pain it caused forced Jackie to listen, turn within, and find the healing that she so desperately needed.

Jackie took the work that we had done to heart. The more she incorporated into her life the things that made her happy, the happier she became. She went through an emotional renaissance of sorts in her later years. I am not sure what happened to Jackie, as we have been out of touch for several years. The last I heard, she was considered a "wild woman" by her neighbors because she was following her dreams and living life according to Jackie. A sharp contrast to the quiet lady who no one used to talk to.

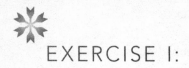

EXERCISE 1:

FUTURE PROGRESSION

This powerful tool for change is often a strong reality check for many of us. After reading this, go to a quiet place and close your eyes. Visualize, imagine, or think about a mirror before you. This is the mirror of prophecy. This magical mirror shows your future based on choices, actions, feelings, and behaviors in your life today. Based on this, it reflects a future you are creating now. What do you see?

_____

_____

_____

_____

_____

Now you are going to visualize your life as it will be once you are healed. Most of us already know exactly how we walk, talk, and live with our pain—but who are you without your disease, anger, addiction, depression, etc., one or five years from now? As you picture this new, healthier reflection of who you are, be specific. Take a moment to imagine . . .

Where are you? What are you wearing? How do you walk? What is the quality of your voice? Who is in your life? What have you achieved? And, most important, how do you feel?

_____

_____

_____

Once you have made contact with this future you, invite her or him to step out of the mirror. Invite your future you to share in this moment and help you to be strong.

Your future you has a job, and that is to help you make choices that are in alignment with the healthy, pain-free, peaceful version of yourself. Notice the contrast between the life you have now and the life you are visualizing that is happy, healthy, and free. This contrast is superimportant. Use it to understand where you are and who you will be. Lean into this future self and invite it to shadow you through these next few weeks of your Convergence Healing. Let it support you and give you strength.

CHAPTER TWO

Give Your Pain a Name

The cure for pain is in the pain.

—Rumi

Pain is the greatest teacher you will ever have. I have said this before and will repeat it, often, because when we finally understand pain's role in healing ourselves, the world will no longer be the big, wounded, spinning ball that it is now.

None of us likes being lectured. None of us likes being told what to do or how to do it, but that is exactly what pain does; it holds us hostage, like the narcissistic boss who demands all our attention and leaves us spent and resentful at the end of a long, hard day.

Pain, when it is left unidentified and unacknowledged, will, quite literally, suck the life energy right out of you.

I know. That is exactly what I let my pain do to me. It will do this to you until you face it.

The pain that I experienced following my accident was a pain that went mostly unrecognized in my household. Both my mother and my father, who were in chronic pain most of their lives, had long ago resigned themselves to using medication and surgery in a futile attempt to manage their pain, and they expected me to do the same. We really did not know any better. We had no awareness of holistic therapies, and the only remedies offered to us were pharmaceuticals and medical interventions.

I grew up in a house where "Don't ask, don't tell" was the unspoken mantra. After my complicated surgery, and even though I lived on crutches for months after I was discharged from the hospital, my parents, to my best recollection, made sure my prescribed medication was available and that was it. They believed that if I took the prescribed pain medications my doctors had ordered, I'd be "fine." Like so many households in that era, it wasn't a concept we talked about. No one thought to ask me what I thought could be done about the pain. Pharmaceuticals were the only option any of us were aware of.

It was as if I had been sworn to keep a big, terrible secret, and so my pain—which was very real, very physical—bonded with my already deep sense of shame. It became a tangible reminder that I was somehow "wrong" and that I was destined never to fit in. So I kept my mouth shut about it. Here I was, a seventeen-year-old who at one minute was launching a professional dancing and acting career, and then the next minute, *bam!* I am hobbling around on crutches in terrific pain, like a worn-out, broken old man. Somehow (I will go into this more in the next chapter) I managed to drag myself along through life, keeping my mouth shut . . . until I just could not do it any longer.

It took a while, but at some point in my twenties I realized that I desperately needed to express my pain or it would eat me alive. So I began casting around, trying to find an outlet, someplace where I could realize and release my pain.

In our culture, we love to share the stories of our pain. Whether we are part of an organized religion or belong to a support group or engage in talk therapy, we are invited into rooms where pain takes center stage. Whether it is the story of a young man who died on a cross for our sins, or it is an AA member telling her story to her peers, or it is a client in a long-term relationship with a psychotherapist, we believe that if we tell our stories to people whom we trust and whom we feel safe with, our pain will somehow vanish.

So I went into therapy. Over the ensuing decade, I spent thousands of dollars and many hours seeing very highly trained, very well-meaning therapists, all of whom expressed deep concern and very focused interest in the story of my pain. I would sit in my therapy sessions telling stories about how much I hurt, and instead of feeling better, I became more and more depressed. There is a saying that goes like this: "You're only as sick as your secrets." Well, it was here that I came to believe you are also as sick as the stories you keep telling yourself.

What I discovered is that by encouraging me to talk about my past experiences—and especially the well-meaning attempts to get me to talk about my accident, which at the time I could not remember completely—the therapists were asking me to stay steeped up to my neck in my own pain.

I was dutiful, I was open, I was committed to the belief that talk therapy would help me out of my pain . . .

But it only made it worse.

So I looked for other places where I could share my pain.

I spent a lot of time in Al-Anon meetings, sharing about my loneliness, my isolation, my "otherness," and, of course, my pain. At first, I felt much better because I was no longer alone. I was finally in a group of people who "got" me. At last! The euphoria I felt at these meetings did not last long, though. I was still me, with my big, dramatic story of having died and come back, of having once danced only to now hobble, to have felt joy that was now buried deep in depression. What I *did* get from my time in Al-Anon was that I needed to get out from under the spell of my own story—once and for all.

The tribe of Al-Anon offered me unconditional love and support, but I soon realized that no group, even this one of very loving souls, could take my pain away.

For some, this kind of sharing is very helpful. But for others, too many others, talking about our pain actually reinforces the prominent place it holds at the center of our identity. Wrapping pain in words can give it too much of the wrong kind of voice. It can give pain a false sense of its own importance and lead it to the bully pulpit from which we shout out to the world who we are. At least, this was true for me.

So what was not working? What was blocking my ability to heal my pain?

LIMITATIONS OF EMPATHY

I began to realize that empathy, specifically empathetic listening, the cornerstone of modern talk therapy, was actually reinforcing my relationship with pain instead of loosening its grip on my body and my aching psyche.

The definition of "empathy" is the ability to "vicariously take on another person's emotions." This is about cultivating the skill to meet another person where he or she lives. That meant that I was engaging with people who were meeting me down in the pit of my despair. These well-meaning, very highly trained people wanted to do this! They wanted to meet me down in the darkness.

But my intuition told me otherwise. What I really needed was to meet someone or connect with something that was on higher ground than I was; I needed to be met with compassion (the recognition of where I am), but I needed a hand up, not a hug from an overly empathetic being.

When I really understood this, I had a breakthrough. Maybe, I began to figure out, just maybe, talking about my pain was not going to help me heal it.

There had to be another way. There had to be a way for me to get past the story my pain loved to tell. There had to be some way I could get past the barricade of words and feelings I had come to associate with my pain. There had to be some way for me to make a clean break.

Then I discovered hypnosis.

THE SILVER BULLET OF PAIN TREATMENT

Hypnosis, according to the Mayo Clinic, a worldwide leader in medical care and research, is a trancelike state in which you practice heightened focus and concentration with the help of a trained therapist or hypnotherapist, or through verbal repetition and/or mental imagery. Contrary to how active meditation and hypnosis are often dramatized as parlor trickery, you do not lose absolute control over your behavior while under its spell. You may not be able to suddenly tap-dance, balance a vase of flowers on your head, or perform a breathtaking rendition of Beethoven's *Moonlight Sonata* on piano. You should remain cognizant, be aware, and remember what happens when you complete the session. However, you should also feel a shift of energy within you, even after a single session. And, especially on the subconscious level, you will begin to be able to approach life differently.

Also known as hypnotherapy or hypnotic suggestion, hypnosis was officially introduced into our modern culture by James Braid, a Scottish surgeon who was an influential pioneer of the treatment. Braid believed that when patients were under the influence of hypnosis, they usually felt calmer and more relaxed. This state can render the patient more open to suggestion. While the term "hypnosis" was coined in the 1840s, healers in ancient China, Egypt, and Greece were practicing the technique, or some form of it, centuries earlier.

A comparative study was published several years ago in *American Health* magazine on the effectiveness of hypnosis. This is what it said: "Psychoanalysis: 38% recovery rate after 600 sessions. Behavior Therapy: 72% recovery rate after 22 sessions. Hypnotherapy: 93% success rate after 6 sessions." And studies are coming in constantly demonstrating the growing recognition that hypnosis is a powerful tool for creating change.

Today, hypnosis is often used to alleviate chronic pain and anxiety, to effectively treat post-traumatic stress disorder (PTSD) and insomnia, to facilitate smoking cessation and weight loss, and to gain control over other addictions, habits, and compulsive behaviors.

When I discovered hypnotherapy, I was studying for my master's degree in consciousness studies. I was studying things like quantum theory, cosmology, the brain-body connection, and the New Thought Movement. I was fascinated by how our thoughts and our feelings affect our DNA, and in my reading, hypnosis and like-minded therapies such as guided imagery, visualization, etc., were mentioned time and time again. So I decided I should learn about them.

But I came to my study of hypnosis with a fair degree of skepticism. I was well into the second month of my hypnosis certification program and was by no means sold on its ability to heal, when, during a practice session, I worked with a fellow student who was having near-debilitating panic attacks. She was desperately trying to get through the course, hold down a job, and deal with her rapidly deteriorating relationship with her parents. I put her in a trance and did some basic relaxation work with her while suggesting that she was protected by a golden shield of light and that any fears and negativity that were around her would simply come into contact with the shield and be dissolved. I told her she could even toss things into the shield if she wanted to and the light and heat from it would burn up anything she gave to it.

I saw her a week later and she was beaming. She told me that she was no longer arguing with her parents and that she had made it through one of the toughest weeks of her life without having a panic attack. She said that she even laughed more that week than she had in years. I was simply amazed. From that moment on I was hooked. If I could help someone make a change like that so effortlessly, then, I found myself wondering, what could I do if I actually put some effort into it for my own symptoms?

Because of this experience, I chose to become a hypnotherapist rather than pursue an MFT (marriage and family therapy) degree. I wanted to help people quickly and effectively move through their pain so that they could immediately begin to live life on a more joyful and fulfilling plane. I knew from my own experience that reliving old traumas and reactivating the traumas that had initially carved deep trenches into a client's neuro-pathways was not necessarily the best treatment strategy. Now I watch miracles almost daily and get to witness my clients go from frozen and stuck to flowing and alive in just a few short sessions.

This is because I see my role as being someone who facilitates the elevation of the vibrations and energies of my clients. I know that I am no good to them if I am only empathizing with them. I believe experiencing empathy is powerful, but emphasizing it as a healing modality isn't as helpful as we have come to think. Why is it helpful to feel the vibration of another person's suffering as your own, and how do we imagine this won't affect us? This is why up to 67 percent of mental health workers are experiencing burnout.

When I was stuck in my own psychologically, emotionally, and physically painful "rock bottom," the last thing I wanted was for my therapist to jump down into that low point to be with me. How would that be helpful? What I wanted and needed was to know that I was going to be able to get out of that dark place, led by the very person holding the light and leading the way. Or, better yet, I needed someone to help me find the confidence and belief in myself to know that I had everything I needed to find my way out of that deep pit myself. What I needed was to know that I could and would help myself. This is what I strive to do for every one of my clients.

This is what hypnosis imparts: the deep truth that the clients have all the tools they need to heal themselves already—that the key to healing lies within.

Hypnotherapy can have qualities of "no mind," which in the Taoist tradition means "no observer." When a person enters a hypnotic state, the mind loses awareness of itself and so the unconscious can be connected with much more easily. This is something quite foreign to most Westerners because we think of thoughtfulness or feeling "out of our mind" as being out of touch. Where hypnosis is concerned, nothing could be further from the truth.

When my clients go into a trance they move into a state of simply being. When we are in pain, whether it is addiction or physical pain, the brain is constantly looking at itself and becomes hyper-aware of its pain. Someone in the throes of addiction sees alcohol everywhere he goes. Someone with back pain is constantly looking for and noticing every twinge and ache and can even project this pain into the future as she anticipates how painful engaging in a particular activity will be. Going into a trance and engaging in the experience of "no mind" helps to relieve pain and gives the brain a new message and a new orientation to pain. When a person enters a state of hypnosis, the body gets to relax. The pain signals can be turned off and our need to pay attention to the pain can be diverted toward something else, allowing the mind to relax too. This is when active healing can take place.

I am still amazed by how quickly the work I do with Convergence Healing can help people release their pain and begin to heal. But I do joke that I if had gone on to become a traditional MFT or LCSW (licensed clinical social worker) instead of getting my MA in consciousness studies, I'd probably be driving a much nicer car!

HEALING WITH HYPNOTIC DIALOGUE

As I mentioned earlier in this chapter, entering into a hypnotic state does not render a person a walking zombie. Hypnosis has been portrayed as being some kind of loony magic trick that is more at home on the Las Vegas Strip than in a healing environment. When a person enters a hypnotic state, she actually can be very aware, present, and attuned to everything that is going on around her. When I use hypnosis with a client, what is actually happening is that we engage in a focused, nonjudgmental, yet very specific dialogue about pain. It is a hard thing to describe, so I am going to show you by letting you in on a session I conducted recently with a woman named Thea.

THEA

I met Thea one warm spring afternoon to see what we could do to help her feel better and release some pain habits. Thea, a wife and mother in her early forties, was a very successful entrepreneur. She had already launched one highly successful company and was now launching another.

Thea told me that every time she achieved any success, she gained weight. Though her weight only fluctuated by twenty pounds, it was enough to mean that she had two closets housing two different sizes and, more important, it meant that Thea became self-conscious and aware of her body in ways that made her uncomfortable. She wanted me to hypnotize her so her weight would stop fluctuating once and for all.

Part of what makes Thea successful is her directness, so after plying me with some delicious snacks, she asked me if, instead of describing to her what our process would be, I would just dive in and "do my thing."

We sat across from each other at an outdoor table, both of us in comfortable chairs. I asked Thea to tell me about her weight. She told me that she had begun putting on weight when she was a girl transitioning into womanhood. She had gone from being a tomboy who spent her time in the outdoors to being the object of too much attention from older boys at school. She also felt that, though her father was very appropriate with her, her mother felt that Thea was "competition" for her husband's attention. When young Thea put on weight, the boys backed off—and so did her mother.

Thea grew up equating having a little bit of extra padding as having an invisible suit of armor; it kept her safe from the unwanted attention of boys and it kept her separate and differentiated from her thin mother. Thea seemed to say everything she needed to say about the weight, so I asked her about that little girl, the young Thea. I was not hearing how the weight was an issue. It helped her in very positive ways, so I probed deeper to better understand what was going on. I was not interested in the details of her stories but in understanding what was actually driving the weight fluctuation itself. I asked Thea to say out loud to her younger self, "I will set you free." When she spoke those words, her whole demeanor changed.

"I will set you free."

I watched as Thea's smiling face gave way to silent tears. I suggested to her that she needed to reassure her younger self that she was safe and that she was in the very capable and loving hands of the now grown Thea. I told her that she no longer had to fight, flee, freeze, or hide—the four classic responses to trauma—and that she could just be. Here. Now. With her grown-up self.

Thea nodded her head and, still weeping, told me that she felt heat radiating from the back of her neck. As she lifted her thick, curly hair, she explained to me that she had just recently been told that her neck was very damaged and that if she did not get treatment for the three vertebrae at the base of her skull, she might one day need surgery. "It feels hot," she said as she stroked the back of her neck. I asked her what she thought might be causing this sensation, and she told me that at the age of six or seven she had been in a terrible auto accident in a car that was being driven by her mother.

"I have never told anyone this story before," she said.

Suddenly, Thea was there again, in the back of an old El Camino, huddled up under the camper top with several of her school friends. Thea was particularly happy because her friends never came to her house to play. She cannot remember where they were going that day, but suddenly her mother, who was driving, yanked the steering wheel and turned the car into the oncoming path of a truck. There was an awful crashing sound, and Thea remembers becoming airborne and bouncing around in the back of the truck with her friends, all of them screaming.

At one point, Thea hit her head so violently on the hard plastic shell of the camper top that her ears rang and her vision blurred. When the car came to a stop, no one spoke a word. Everyone was too stunned.

Within seconds, it seemed, a police officer was at the driver's-side window, questioning Thea's mother about what had happened. Then Thea, who knew she had injured her neck, listened as her mother lied to the law.

At that moment, Thea knew that she had to keep her mouth shut to protect her mother (back then, she thought her mother might go to jail if the officer knew the truth and, now with hindsight, knowing that her mother was a longtime addict, she knew that she very well may have) and to make the awful ordeal less traumatic for her friends. It was a double-loaded, very big lie for someone so young to carry within her, and it was now finally showing up as a very serious neck injury.

Thea blurted out, "I get it! This isn't about my weight at all; it's about the accident. The lie. My voice. I lost my singing voice and my voice of telling the truth. I lost my voice because I went along with the lie."

In a moment of crystalline recognition, Thea told me that she finally understood what it had cost her to hide her own injuries and the truth. It was a complex wound that had gone "underground" for most of her life. She had had to live with her mother's emotional abandonment and her unacknowledged injury her whole life. Now it was here, out in the open. The very competent and emotionally available adult Thea had unearthed it.

We took a short break and drank some water. We chatted briefly about what she had learned. "Not being able to trust my mom was overwhelming for me." I nodded in agreement. I asked her about her neck. "If I can heal it . . . maybe I can sing again!" Thea's face lit up.

We were not quite there. The occurrence of an unexpected connection, this complaining of a particular problem when the root of an issue is really something else, was something that we needed to follow.

I asked Thea if she wanted to go a little deeper and get to know this pain more intimately so she could come up with an action plan for healing it. "Yes! Of course! Let's do it!" she said with a smile.

Even though she had just touched on one of the most traumatic and influential events of her life (which was spoken of for the first time), she remained calm, open, and present: this is the active healing state that hypnosis facilitates. It creates a state of energized calm that allows a person to go deep without disrupting the serene energy that healing generates.

We moved inside, away from the late-afternoon shadows, and

Thea lay down on her couch. Seated in a chair at her feet, I led her through a classic relaxation technique that allowed her to acknowledge the external world—her dog kept bringing us toys and the laundry was noisily spinning in the next room—and then to shift her gaze by rolling her eyes to the back of her head and closing them. This would naturally draw her gaze inward. We "scanned" her body by bringing awareness to each of her body parts, beginning with her feet and moving up toward her head. When we got to her neck, I asked Thea if she associated any feeling or color or sound with that part of her body. I asked her too if it had a name, or if she wanted to name it. "It's Theo," she said with a little laugh.

"Okay, Thea. Let's get to know Theo and find out what he needs," I said.

As Thea lay on the couch with her eyes closed and her hands gently crossed over her heart, we began. I asked her to allow herself to dissolve into the present moment, to just give her body up to the current of stillness that was surrounding her.

The more relaxed she became, the more aware Thea grew of some really interesting sensations in her neck. At one point, she even said she felt like it was "gurgling" as though it were trying to speak. We talked then about how, when pain is recognized, it releases vital energy that has been pent up, and the sensations of this can be surprising. When I do this with my clients, this energy can come out in all kinds of ways, from tremors to major shaking to coughs, itches, fidgeting, sneezes, and gurgling stomachs.

Before we could address the pain directly, I asked Thea to tell her pain four things—and I ask each of my clients to do the same. I asked her to tell her pain:

Thank you.

I love you.

I am sorry.

Forgive me.

When we honor our pain with this mantra of acknowledgment, we liberate it from our ego and our conscious mind, the mind that has been deeply invested in holding on to that pain at all costs.

I watched as Thea spoke these words, and then the energy around her changed. Suddenly the room was charged. "Something just shifted!" she said, eyes still closed and a broad smile across her face. "Pain is trapped energy, Thea. You are releasing it now," I told her. With that release, we were ready to step into the final part of our session.

I asked Thea if she could identify what Theo needed on a physical level (the body) to heal. "To be touched," she said. What does he need on an emotional level? "He needs my attention," she said. What does he need on the level of spirit? "To sing again, like when I was little, before the accident!" (This was the third time she had mentioned singing.)

"Can you provide those things?" Thea began to explain that she did not have enough time or money. That her kids and her husband already did not get enough of her attention. That they were saving for . . . I gently interrupted her and brought her attention back to Theo. I pointed out that perhaps her thinking might be flawed, because, in truth, there is all the time in the world for healing.

Often we think we have to devote enormous amounts of time to these requests that come from the pain, but I have discovered that the length of time you spend engaging in a particular request is far less important than actually doing it. Thea could find time to sing throughout her day, and just because the pain requested her to take a class for singing, it did not necessarily have to be for the rest of her life. Her family would understand if she needed to take care of this old injury. Perhaps they would even be grateful that she did.

I suggested that there is always money for self-care, for true healing, if we really want to feel better. When you set your mind to something or decide it's time to heal, it is amazing how that experience simply comes to you. I suggested that she might need to come up with a mantra to remind herself that she and she alone was responsible for Theo's care.

"There is so much time. I have so much money. I just have to spend it!" Thea blurted this out. It took even me by surprise. We both laughed, hard.

"Where did that come from?" she asked, smiling.

"It is your unconscious telling you that you have everything you need to support and heal Theo," I said.

Now it was time for her to look at what her pain specifically needed on the physical, emotional, and spiritual levels.

"Reiki. Theo needs Reiki," Thea said without missing a beat. Reiki is a modern, holistic understanding of the ancient tradition of the "laying on of hands." It is a highly spiritual practice not associated with any religion and a fantastic tool to combine with other healing modalities, from allopathic to alternative. The idea is that the practitioner feels life-force energy (also known as chi, qi, or Kundalini) and guides it into and through the body to promote the flow of healing.

"What kind of emotional support does he need?" I asked.

"Theo needs me to love and respect him and to acknowledge him," Thea responded.

"What kind of spiritual support can you give him?" was my last question.

"He needs to sing. I need to give him singing lessons."

Thea was a woman after my own heart.

With those words, I gently encouraged Thea to bring her awareness back to the room around her. She opened her eyes and smiled. Her healing had begun. I asked her if she did these things—sing, Reiki, change and challenge her perception of money, really get to know Theo and listen and respect him—would she feel better? She excitedly agreed, as the healing was already in motion. She had her mantra—"There is so much time and money. I just need to spend it!"—and a concrete plan of action to heal her wounded neck.

HOW OUR PAIN FOOLS US

Thea's story is so important because it shows us a fundamental truth about pain: it is elusive and it is quite the trickster. Thea was certain her discomfort, her pain, was caused by her weight gain. In fact, her weight gain was just another symptom of a deeper, earlier wound that had gone unhealed. Thea is a very aware and intuitive person, so she knew that what she needed to address had happened to her younger self, and yet she was truly amazed at how swiftly our hypno-conversation had moved her through her thoughts about weight—and the pattern of gaining and then losing weight that had begun in her adolescence—and right to the true source of her pain.

This is the trap of partial awareness that most of us fall into despite our best intentions, because pain loves to shape-shift. Pain

GIVE YOUR PAIN A NAME

is designed to "disguise" itself so that it can keep us under its thrall. It does not help that we are not encouraged to turn and face it and actually befriend it. You will see, as you make your way through this book, that facing your pain and letting it guide you is the path to true healing. And within a couple of months Thea dropped her extra weight. She naturally stopped overeating as soon as she began singing and receiving healing touch therapy on her neck.

EXERCISE II:

CREATE YOUR MANTRA OR METAPHOR

Creating a positive mantra helps set your intention for health. Repeating positive thoughts to yourself is cleansing and energizing.

For example, I think of my mantra as my mission statement:

"My purpose is to bring healing to all aspects of my life, and in doing so, to share that healing with others so that they may heal, too."

Or, more simply, "I am well. I bring wellness into the world."

"I am loved by the universe."

"I welcome abundance and live my life with grace and ease."

"The universe loves me."

Or, "I commit to living in the moment, taking full responsibility for me and embracing the power that comes with freeing any sense of victimhood."

Try to let go of all expectations and ask yourself: How do I want to feel? Develop a mantra that feels really personal and right for you. It may feel awkward to use it at first, but pretty quickly you'll find it will give you a quick blast of energetic love. If at first your mantra feels inauthentic, that is simply because it is unfamiliar.

Revise and practice saying your mantra until the words truly become you.

If you are still feeling stuck in crafting your very own mantra, feel free to borrow a favorite:

"I release and let go of everyone and everything, conscious and subconscious, that is out of alignment with my highest potential."

CHAPTER THREE

Step out of the Fog

Keep all your attention in the present moment—refrain from living in the past or worrying about the future. Learn to trust what you cannot see far more than what you can see.

—Caroline Myss

"Jarring" is the word I use most often to describe my deadly accident. Unlike a lot of the happily-ever-after stories we hear about people who have had near-death experiences, my own brush with death had the opposite effect on me.

My encounter with the bearded messenger from the other side did not ignite in me a passion for living; instead, the overwhelming impact of that crash broke me up on so many levels that my fragile ego caved beneath a staggering sense of shame. With that shame came a kind of paralysis that rendered me unable to speak my truth, feel love, or move around the world in ways that felt authentic and meaningful to me. I was a dancer no longer, so who was I?

Instead of having some kind of emotional or spiritual epiphany that transcended all the pain I experienced in that one horrific, life-altering moment, I became my pain.

I survived, but I lost my ability to live independent of my pain. Instead of coming out of the wreckage with a clearer sense of purpose and belonging, I emerged crippled by a sense of being "wrong" in the world that rendered me wounded, confused, sad, and unsure of myself.

So I found myself living in a state of trauma-induced fogginess that left me lost and lonely and groping in darkness just beyond love's reach for years and years. And years.

My pain, like Thea's, went into deep, deep hiding. It went so far underground, so far beyond my own messed-up adolescent consciousness, that it began to control me, like a sadistic puppeteer. I came to from that accident doped up by depression, shame, unexpressed rage, and all kinds of toxic fallout that kept me locked up and living a lie for many years to come.

It took me a long time to find my way out of that deep fog, and I learned the hard way that we cannot heal, on any level, as long as we stay lost within the blinding haze of our pain.

I woke up in the hospital after my accident, my worried parents peering down on me with expressions on their faces that I interpreted as "What have you done now?" rather than "How can we help you?" My knee was so messed up that the doctors decided they would bandage me up and send me home; then, when the tissue around my wound was healed enough, they would bring me back in to perform surgery on me.

The day after the accident, I left the hospital looking like a mummy who had been forgotten halfway through the embalming process. I remember feeling so naked and exposed as I was pushed out of the hospital in a wheelchair, draped only in an ill-fitting hospital gown and shivering under a thin blanket, my left leg mummified at a forty-five-degree angle, encased in a hard cast that ran hip to toe. My right hand, my dominant hand, was buried deep in a cast that ran down to the tip of my fingers. I could not walk, write, feed myself, or get dressed, so once I was home, I was basically propped up on our sofa, naked except for the hard white shrouds covering my limbs.

On top of the indignity of all these physical limitations, no one ever once asked me what happened after my feeble explanation that I had been blinded by a car's headlights. They did not seem to be concerned that there had been a big car behind me, a car that had come so close that I was blinded by its headlights as they burned into my side-view mirrors. For them, the simple explanation was enough and it was never spoken of again.

There were no questions about how the accident had happened, why someone had been driving that close to me, or who had hit me. Part of me was grateful that they did not ask, but the majority of me felt resentful that they did not pursue the person who had done this. Had they asked, I would have had to tell them about my dying and getting kicked out of heaven, and that was not something I wanted to tell anyone. They were just happy I was alive, and I guess that was all that mattered.

Why had the driver not stopped? Why did I feel that the person who had tailgated me that night was someone I knew, someone who wished me harm (but who was someone I could not identify)?

How could I tell them that I had died and that, now that I was back, I did not know how to live?

It was clear that I was badly hurt, but unbeknownst to them—

and to me—the worst injury I suffered was to my brain. The impact of that crash—the jarring—had sent my mind off on a self-punishing course that would take me decades to free myself from. The only way my confused psyche knew how to handle the undiagnosed brain trauma I suffered was to go numb.

After a week and a half at home, I went back to the hospital to have my knee rebuilt. As I mentioned earlier in the book, this surgery was so new, so experimental, that other orthopedic surgeons were brought in from around the country to observe it. What I remember most about the experience is how ignored I was—as a human being—as the surgeon in charge of my case talked to everyone in that operating room as though I was not even there. It was as though my knee had wandered in on its own, unattached to a boy's body, a boy who was being swallowed whole by confusion and shame.

Then there was the anesthesiologist, who appeared at the head of the operating table. He slipped a mask over my face and began, in a mocking voice, to sing, "Go to sleep, go to sleep, little baby..." as though I were an infant with no sense of self. I was appalled. I remember a dark rage rising within me, but then everything, including myself, went into black and ... when I awoke, all of the scalding anger that had risen in me just before I went unconscious was now locked into my delicately stitched-up body.

I was sent home, achy and on crutches after three days in the hospital, and it would be another five months before I was well enough to leave the house and go back to school.

It was my senior year, the year that is supposed to be the apotheosis of one's youth. But I was such a late bloomer. The hiding of my sexuality had stunted me emotionally and I never had the opportunity to rebel, to have a high school crush, or to disobey my parents and find my true self. I spent so much of my time being and doing what I was supposed to be and do that I was losing sight of who I really was, and now I was even more dependent on my parents at a time when that was the last thing I really wanted.

Now I was hobbling back into school with a leg brace that had steel rods that went from my crotch area down to my lower calf. This would stabilize my knee so that I could walk with a crutch or a cane. Unfortunately, the bullies were lying in wait.

It took only three days for the attack to happen. I was gimping down a long hallway, trying to not be late to my next class, when someone kicked my crutches right out from under me. There I was, flattened on the floor, being laughed at. No one stopped to help me, and I hit the ground smack in the middle of my left kneecap. (The surgery had been on the back of my left knee.) Shock waves of pain, fear, and embarrassment reverberated through me as I struggled to get up and retrieve my crutches. But that one awful incident was it.

After that, everyone seemed to give me the widest berth possible. I seesawed between raw humiliation and utter loneliness until I graduated a few months later. I focused all the energy I could on acting as if nothing was wrong. I never knew why the bullying stopped until I attended my ten-year high school reunion. There, a friend from back in our junior high days named Rob told me that he had informed my bullies that if they messed with me again they would be answering to him next. Rob, who was a jock himself, had swooped in and come to my defense like a silent guardian angel. I wish I had known that sooner! My sense of myself as a victim was so raw back then; I lived in a chronic state of anxiety about when the next ambush would come. I had spent ten years—ten years!—carrying around the fear of those high school bullies.

I felt something so dark being released that night when Rob told me what he had done; immediately my sense of shame eased up and I looked around that room at my long-ago classmates and for the first time I did not feel threatened. I hugged Rob and thanked him profusely, not at all able to explain what a gift his connection had given me. I was filled with a nearly overwhelming sense of gratitude for that one spontaneous random act of kindness he had shown me.

But I did not feel such gratitude back when I was a disabled seventeen-year-old. Instead, I began to become mired in the terrible quicksand of the "Don't ask, don't tell" message I had gotten from the moment I came to in the hospital, following my crash. No one, not my parents, my doctors, or any adults in my life, seemed to want to know what had happened that fateful night. My family would ask me how I was doing, but I felt that they really did not want to know. I could not tell them that I thought about suicide daily and that I felt lost, frightened, and confused.

My pain had nowhere to go. I was not encouraged to talk about my experience, and I certainly was not encouraged to ask for help. The expectation was that I would simply "man up," stay the course, follow doctors' orders, and get through the ordeal as quickly and as quietly as possible.

I had no idea of the price I would pay for maintaining this kind of unhealthy silence as my young life progressed.

Somehow, despite the many months of school I had missed, I managed to graduate on time. I even tried to dance again around the end of the first summer after high school, but I pushed myself way too hard, way too fast, and injured myself again. I took this "failure" to be a sure sign that I would never dance again. I also left home that summer and went to a special program at San Francisco

State. By then, my energy was defined by a near-permanent state of feeling utterly defeated about almost everything in life. I became more and more isolated as I kept trying, in vain, to gain some sort of control over my life. It did not help that I just did not like the energy of San Francisco; it was too much of a party town for me.

Since the accident, I had been in a constant state of anxiety, on top of still being in a lot of physical pain, so I bailed on San Francisco and came home and enrolled at San Jose State University. I stayed, head down, and after two years I transferred into a program at California State University at Northridge. I studied humanities with a theater emphasis. I had decided to be an actor, since this was something I knew I could do well. I lasted only a year at CSUN; I felt disappointed by the program I had enrolled in and I was struggling to fit in socially and to have normal relationships with people my own age.

While I was there, I toyed with the idea of "coming out," but I was too frightened to do it. Instead, I got involved with a young woman I really liked and respected. However, not long after I began a relationship with her, I had my first gay sexual experience with a man that I did not like or respect or even find attractive. I looked at this as a test. It was clear what this man wanted from me, and so I figured that if I slept with him and liked having sex with a man whom I did not even find attractive, then I had to be gay. Well, I did like it, and the fact that I liked it scared me so much that I immediately slammed that door shut and stayed in my relationship with the woman.

For most of that year, we lived together, and when she got pregnant the suppressed constant state of panic I had been living in really hit a new height. I was not naturally suited to be in a sexual relationship with a woman, though I still was not prepared to admit this to myself. I knew that I certainly was not prepared to be a father, given how inauthentic and not even present in the world I felt. When she decided to have an abortion, it took a great toll on us both; it brought our relationship to an end and it propelled me to finally own up to who I was.

That summer, I came out. I also moved back to San Jose and reenrolled at San Jose State University. I was ping-ponging through my life, but at least I was no longer hiding an essential truth about myself—not to myself anyway. I went into a period of being celibate and focused on my studies. I did not have another gay sexual experience until I had my first boyfriend, when I was twenty-two. I was with Steve for about a year, and yet I still had not told my family that I was gay. That would not happen for another year.

Being in a relationship with a man (even a dysfunctional one) did help me deal with the shame I had felt my whole life over the fact that I was born gay. I tried to see a therapist, but it was incredibly expensive (and I had no money in my twenties). Also, many therapists back then tried to talk people out of being gay. I knew this approach was not for me because I had already been trying to talk myself out of being gay for my whole life! So what I did was read books about growing up gay and joined an organization called Parents and Friends of Lesbians and Gays (PFLAG). I made a point of speaking with quite a few parents about what it was like for them to have gay children, so I could get a sense of what my parents might experience once I came out to them.

One of the fantastic things PFLAG taught me was to look at the fact of being gay as a gift, not a shortcoming. I'd heard from Steve and the few friends who knew I was gay that here I had been given this great gift, but I wanted to throw it in the trash. Was I gay? I related to and was attracted to both men and women, so maybe I was bisexual. It took a long time to just relax around who I was and just be. I started to appreciate and love this middle sex that I was. Along with this new self-acceptance, the physical pain started to lessen (although I was not consciously aware of the connection) and become more manageable, and the fog began, finally, to lift a little.

Armed with this new sense of warmth, feeling, and understanding that I had gained from PFLAG, I decided to finally face my fears and come out to my parents. I gathered a bunch of books, pamphlets, and a video for my "coming out" box. I also wrote a long letter to my parents and I put that in the box too. Then I gift-wrapped it in paper I hand painted. I honestly felt like I was giving my parents the best gift possible: the truth of who I was.

Unfortunately, my parents did not quite see it that way. They loved me but they did not want me to be gay. They had invested so much time and energy in refusing to see who I truly was that their initial response was one of anger. I was breaking the family rule of "Don't ask, don't tell," and they did not like it.

Despite their reaction, I felt better. The care I had taken in preparing for this moment had been, I see, a way of preparing my soul to handle a less-than-loving reaction. I realized that I finally loved myself enough to want to package my truth as a beautiful gift.

My parents reacted just as I had thought they would. They were disappointed. I assume they felt cheated. But I did not. I felt liberated—guilty for making them feel bad, but liberated. When I left them, I felt strong and I noticed that the stars seemed to be shining more brightly in the vast sky. I had put such care and thought into the gift I was giving my parents that my soul experienced a deep moment of cathartic release.

This experience led me, naturally, to ask myself some important questions. Questions that I had been too shut down, too repressed, to even formulate before. These questions included:

What had I been so afraid of?
Could I still be loved even if I was not understood?
Would I still love even if I was not understood?

I had been afraid that I would never be loved. I learned the day I came out to my parents that love does not work like that. My parents did love me. They just were really upset about what they understood as homosexuality and what that meant to them about who I was. They had to now deal with their own issues of shame, anger, and embarrassment. I could accept that! But what about me? Would I be capable of loving someone who did not "get" or want to "get" me? I realized, given how fiercely I loved my parents, the answer was a resounding yes.

Love was the answer.

The fog continued to clear with this understanding.

While going through the coming-out process was a long and arduous experience for me, finally being open, honest, and up-front about my sexuality helped me gain strength and perspective, and I found that I wanted to face other parts of my life that needed fixing. This *one positive action* was a huge step in the right direction for me. It is true what they say: the first step is always the hardest. Once you have taken it, you have established some momentum and direction and so the next step is easier, and before you know it, you are actually taking decisive steps away from your pain and your shame and moving toward your life and love.

But you have to take that first big step. You have to be honest with yourself and those around you about who you really are.

The process of coming out gave me the strength and the insight to understand that there are things in life I would be able to change and things I would not. Some people would meet my truth with warmth and delight, others would meet my truth with detached acceptance, and still others would meet my truth with hate. I was really starting to understand that I could handle all of these reactions as long as I stayed honest and loving with myself.

Acceptance. That was a huge, huge lesson. I began to understand that I would remain in physical, emotional, and spiritual pain as long as I did not accept myself. Once I made some peace with myself, it was a revelation to realize that I now had a greater capacity to accept others. Tolerance was pretty good medicine. Acceptance was *really* good medicine. Love, unconditional, openhearted love, was the *best* medicine. Love was the way to defeat pain. Love was the one thing that would finally burn away the fog.

After my first boyfriend and I broke up, I found myself tumbling back into a depression, and further and further from the free-spirited dancer I had been before the crash. I had to do something. While coming out had alleviated some of it, I was still in dire emotional and physical pain and had to find my way out of the unbearable haze of the half a life that I was living. Either that, or I would die, a lonely young man who had experienced his life only as an outsider, as a victim.

Most of my twenties were spent living from paycheck to paycheck, being in dysfunctional relationships, and existing in a state of full-on survival mode. I wanted to stop being victimized by my pain, but I did not know how. Everyone thought I was happy and a "survivor," but behind the mask I was a wreck and barely getting by. Plus, based on my circumstances, I felt that there was no time or money to spend on healing. I struggled with everything: keeping a roof over my head, putting food in my body (the importance of healthy food had not been widely realized yet), and getting enough rest. Every day was an exercise in nail-biting scarcity. It was no way to live.

This was all I knew. I had grown so comfortable being in pain that I could not even see that I used it as an excuse for why I was not happier, more successful, or more fulfilled. I did not know how to be without all the shame-filled negative beliefs about myself I had held so dear for so long. I clung to my shame like it was a life raft, even as my health plummeted.

As I moved into my thirties, fear was still rotting my insides, while externally things started to look up. I had a bit of a career and a mildly steady relationship, and I bought my first house. As things started to settle for me both emotionally and spiritually, I had brief glimpses of what a life without shame or pain could be like, and so I knew that this hateful numbness I could not shake was not the only way to be in the world. Still, I just could not break free; I could not become un-numb.

After I ended my third abusive relationship, and while I was working two jobs and suffering from such severe sciatica that I could barely walk, a friend gave me the number of an acupuncturist. I would regularly throw my back out due to my not properly taking care of myself physically, not being able to deal with the emotional wounds that seemed locked into my body, and the physical fact that because of my leg being rebuilt I had one leg shorter than the other. I literally scuttled like a crab with my belly facing skyward into his office, but after that first session I actually walked out of his office upright. I was able to put one foot in front of the other for the first time in weeks. I was still in some pain, but I left feeling a warm energy coursing through my body. That visit was transforming. It began my journey into alternative therapies.

As much as seeing my cousin perform in *How to Succeed in Business Without Really Trying* when I was nine made me want to be a performer, realizing what an acupuncturist could achieve in only one session had me hooked on holistic healing. My appetite had been whetted and I needed to know more. Could it be true? Could I actually hope to be healed? All I knew was that I wanted, badly, to find out.

At first this desire felt overwhelming. It *was* overwhelming, but little by little, tiny step by tiny step, I began to commit to a new awareness about my wants, my needs, and my pain. I had not been honest with myself about how much pain I was in. I had to cop to my pain first and recognize how lousy my life really was. Any thoughts that my pain was okay or helping me in any way were now dashed. I could no longer hide it. I was in pain.

As I began to acknowledge and embrace with compassion the victim that I had become, I began to grow into the man that I was meant to be. It was like I decided to reach down and give myself a hand up. Maybe the man that I was meant to be could help the pathetic soul that I was and guide me out of what misery my life had become. I was recognizing that I had the power to help myself.

When I stopped being the victim of all the things that I thought life had done to me and I simply accepted them as some facts in the much larger story of me, things began to change. The grip of the drama I had created with my pain finally began to loosen. My mind began to feel free and my heart began to hope.

After the acupuncture, I tried every holistic therapy I could find and afford to pay for. Several years later I discovered Rolfing. With just one session, I felt another layer of the fog lift. Finally, I was able to actually remember the moment of impact of the accident. This key moment in my life had been buried deep within my unconscious for almost thirty years.

Rolfing, also known as Structural Integration, is a type of bodywork that focuses on the connective tissue. As a massage therapist focuses on certain muscles, the Rolfer focuses on ligaments, tendons, and cartilage. She was working on my injured knee when I had a sudden flash of memory.

I was back at the scene of the accident and saw that I did not have time to do anything to save myself. In that moment and for several days afterward, I slowly started to forgive myself for not being able to prevent the accident from happening. I realized, finally, that I had done nothing wrong. The missing piece of my memory and the experience of dying had been exhumed, and I felt almost whole.

The brain trauma I experienced from being slammed into the semitruck had gone undiagnosed until I started to work with a healer who used neuro-feedback to bring relief to her clients with PTSD and behavioral disorders. My brain patterns showed a very clear trauma and recovery pattern. Under her expert care, all those years of feeling like I was walking in a fog, being frustrated for no apparent reason, having mood swings, and literally substituting words—I would think one word but say another—finally made some sense to me. If nothing else, the clarity of realizing what was actually going on in my brain really helped unbury my pain. It was awesome to discover that my brain had a plasticity to it that allowed it to heal.

Since I was beginning to step up and take responsibility for my life, it occurred to me that maybe now I no longer needed blame as a life strategy, but I had put a lot of stock in it. Why did I feel the need to blame the phantom driver of the car that hit me for my pain? If I kept blaming whoever it was, it was like I was still looking into those side-view mirrors that had blinded me so many years before.

Today, now that I have been able to forgive the driver of the car that hit me and have forgiven myself for enabling my own pain for so long, I "see" the accident even more clearly. The well-rehearsed feelings and well-worn stories about the event that I used to tell myself no longer trigger knee-jerk anger or bitterness and they steal less and less of my time. As my emotional wounds heal, my mind and heart relax and my physical body continues to heal. I now work hard to fill with love the space that my pain once occupied.

I have had so many friends, loved ones, and even clients say, "It must have been hard to forgive the driver that hit you." It was. For a very long time, it was impossible.

I was not going to be anything—not a dancer, not a decent romantic partner, not a contributing member of any community—if I held on to all of that blame and my identity as a victim. I had to forgive the driver in order to move on and grow beyond the long shadow cast on my life by that accident. Once I realized that blame was controlling my life, it became easy for me to forgive the driver. And my parents. And my less-than-perfect exes. And myself. Especially myself. I wanted healing, not harm.

Letting go of blame means that those of us suffering a form of pain will have to turn and face our misery, anger, frustration, and fear head-on. The fault might not be ours, but this is the one life we have, and lifting this veil on our own behaviors will turn up the volume on our first step of healing: awareness. The mental space we create by cleaning out and removing all need for blame leaves room for more prosperous beliefs to become a part of our consciousness.

As we leave blame and enter responsibility, our thinking becomes clearer. The road out of suffering becomes apparent.

Like so many, I'd also suffered with depression for years without knowing it. I realize now that another of my strategies for surviving was just to push through (sound familiar?). Perhaps, like your parents, this is what my parents had taught me to do. They are fighters, and they don't give up. While I am so grateful they taught me that, now I realize that there is a massive difference between being stoic and being strong: one comes at great cost to your health while the other pays beautiful dividends. This is a distinction I am still learning and am grateful to share with you now, as I do with my clients.

As more and more clarity began to take shape in my life, I realized that in order to break free of my deadening fog I had to first recognize it for what it was. At the heart of living in chronic pain was radical self-denial. On almost every level, my life was a lie. The fog, for me—and I have come to learn for my clients and the millions of the rest of us who are hobbled by pain—was denial: denial of who I am, denial of my need to be free and happy, denial that I am human and easily wounded and harmed.

A child who fakes or exaggerates fear or pain receives attention. She understands early on that being "the victim" pays off. The heroin addict benefits from shooting up by getting to temporarily forget his problems. The writer crippled by anxiety benefits from being anxious by not having to turn in a screenplay and risk being judged. The family martyr benefits from taking care of everyone else and not having to focus on herself.

When our strategies for dealing with our pain are all about deadening it, there is a short-term payoff; but over the long term, denial of our true pain will make us sick on every level.

So the fog creeps in and it gets thicker, and deeper, and colder, and if we do not turn and face it, it will envelop us and become us. Stepping out of the fog takes a lot of courage and a lot of guts because the pull of the familiar can be so irresistible, like the sirens from mythology that call out seductively from the rocks, trying to lure lost sailors to their death. We have to resist the call and magnetic pull of the familiar, the habitual, the deadening, and take action. This is not easy, but you're here with me now, so we both know it's possible.

I had to learn to stop denying, and instead I had to identify all the positive intentions I had that were actually enabling my pain. Before I recognized the patterns that I was stuck in and discovered my true course to healing, I just blamed everything on my accident (and a few Hollywood casting directors). It was always someone else's fault. My victim loved pointing a finger, and whenever the going got tough for me, he reared his pathetic head.

After my accident, first I isolated myself, which really gave me the chance to build up my inner victim. Then, when I did want to be in relationships, I chose people who needed more fixing than I did. That way, the focus was always off me. With little to no sense of self-worth, I consistently created environments where I could avoid confronting what truly ailed me. While the world was out there waiting for me, I felt safe and limited within the confining gates of what I knew. I had to get wounded over and over again before I finally had enough and realized I had to get honest with myself and meet my pain head-on.

Moving past our pain is made even harder when the people around us, however unintentionally, often benefit from our staying in a state of pain. We humans tend to identify ourselves by how we orient ourselves to one another, and so we rely on pretty broad ideas about who others are to reinforce our own sense of self. I had been a martyr to pain for so long that most of the people in my life did not react very well when I started to shed my victim role. This is because my changing meant that they might have to change, even if it just meant they needed to update their ideas about who I was.

So when you make the commitment to step out of the fog, you have to really make a commitment to yourself and trust that you can undertake this journey under your own steam. You have to really begin to trust that you are—*you* are—your own best healer. You have to be patient. Healing is a journey—it is a series of actions. To begin, it takes just one small step and a giant amount of commitment and perseverance. Like all journeys, it is a lot of "one step forward, two steps back." It is like a new dance that you are learning for the first time. Approach this awesome journey with the love and respect you would bring to the dance floor for your first thrilling lesson. Let yourself learn the steps and thrive. It is the only way.

My own healing took quite some time, but not nearly as much time as it took for me to embed myself in the dark, cold fog of victimhood. Sure, I was broken up pretty badly in that car accident, but so what? I was still alive. I just had to learn how to live.

Once I began to turn my intentions around and really learned to name my pain, good things began to happen. I found that the more honest and willing I became, the release of pain brought a cascade of healing into other areas of my life. For example, it is quite common for me to see a client who is having digestive issues, and as we work on those issues, the client will notice that his or her personal relationships improve. A cigarette smoker stops smoking and his anger levels go down. A pot smoker stops smoking weed and her creativity shoots up. When we are lost in the fog, we tend to stay focused on numbing our pain and lose sight of the fact that our pain is within us and it is connected to every aspect of our lives.

The concept of stepping out of the fog will take time, dedication, and delicacy, but one positive step in the right direction followed by another always kept me on the path toward my own Convergence Healing. Your pain and the chaos it creates concealing itself must be revealed for what it truly is. This is the only way to burn off the fog.

I had to commit to knowing who I really was, as opposed to who I thought I was, in order to begin to heal. I had to ask myself tough, honest questions. Was I okay with living in a state of chronic fear and pain? Was I willing to do the work required to heal? Did I want to spend another minute of my time shaming myself? Was I really going to live a healthy, pain-free life if I kept hiding who I actually was?

HOW TO NAVIGATE OUT OF YOUR FOG

How do you navigate your way out of the fog? If you are suffering in a fog of fear, pain, shame, and the unknown and are hoping to discover a clearer path to your best health possible, you need to:

- **Stop denying your pain.** Stand in your truth and take absolute responsibility for your health as it is today. With as little emotion as possible, identify the plain facts of your situation.
- **Release any sense of feeling sorry for yourself.** Decide that you will no longer be the victim to your pain.

- **Stop blaming yourself, others, or the circumstances of your life (the story) for your pain.** Blame is the enemy of true health and healing.

- **Learn to forgive yourself and you will begin to forgive others.** This will unlock the prison of your pain. One powerful tool is the Hawaiian forgiveness prayer, which focuses on total responsibility for our lives and all the experiences within it. It's called *ho'oponopono*. Joe Vitale translated this longer ritual into a simple mantra: "I love you, I'm sorry, please forgive me, and thank you." You can say this to yourself and to others. It is a powerful tool.

- **Love, love, love!** Do things that are good for you, mind, body, and spirit. Nurture yourself and make life choices that cultivate love, not hurt. So, if your instinct is to numb out with TV, wine, Internet browsing, or another vice, instead give yourself a foot rub, go for a walk, or turn on music and dance around the house. Whatever will redirect you into love, do that.

- **Be mindful of how you think.** I work constantly on redirecting my thoughts. When I realize that I'm obsessing or lapsing into blame, I consciously choose to think instead about how I can better love and care for myself. Our thoughts have the power to heal us. The mind can serve us or break us. You've got to train it to serve you.

- **Chant, "Faith, not fear!"** The brain cannot be in faith and fear at the same time. It is impossible. Even split seconds where you can forget your pain can help you find cracks of light in the darkness.

ISABELLA

When Isabella came to me to do some work on herself, I was flattered. She is a highly respected healer in her own right, a career coach, a yoga master, a corporate speaker, and a teacher. It was a personal reminder that even we healers need support, and I was honored that Isabella had chosen to work with me.

There was a familiarity to Isabella's story that intrigued me. It was not the story itself, although there were commonalities, but the "fog" that blinded her from being able to heal. Isabella had been walking around in her own personal fog even after all the healing work she had done on herself and with thousands of clients. It was a classic experience of not being able to see the forest for the trees.

Isabella was a diabetic, seriously overweight, and at a loss as to why she constantly ate things that wreaked havoc with her body. She was "cheating" constantly and felt that she had very little control over her sweet tooth. This upset her deeply, as she knew she was harming herself, but restricting the foods she ate felt like depravation and not eating sweets and junk food felt like punishment. After all, sweets were what lifted her spirits when she was struggling. Yes, even we healers have our bad days. (This is usually how and why many of us became healers in the first place.)

As we explored Isabella's life we discovered that "it was never about the food." For Isabella, being fat was a way of punishing herself and restricting love. Deep down inside, Isabella felt that she did not deserve to be loved. She discovered that her being overweight "spoke to how unaccepted I felt as a kid. Overweight has been the prison of my self-abandonment."

As a child, Isabella got the unspoken message that she was there for others and not for herself. She was abused and bullied, and had an alcoholic father and a disappointed mother. There was a lot of chaos and pain. In the work we did together, we discovered that Isabella was holding on to a lot of anger for not being able to heal her father and being overly focused on pleasing her mother.

Isabella realized her weight gain was tied to her feeling lost in the world. The extra pounds literally grounded her. Her weight issues did not come on until Isabella was in her midthirties, and the diabetes did not develop until her midforties. She had lost her role as a go-between for her parents and she quite literally did not know what to do or how to be in the world. Overly sensitive, she judged herself by her outward appearance and other people's standards. Her downward cycle easily perpetuated itself. Food became her way of "crying on the inside," her coping mechanism. Isabella was still living her life for everyone else and the weight and diabetic issues were forcing her to begin loving herself.

As each revelation hit her, Isabella started to treat herself a little better. She discovered that she was ignoring her core self and only functioning at half capacity. What she wanted more than anything was to be an actor. As years went by it became harder and harder for her to perform. Self-criticism and the literal weight from the past were always paralyzing her. At the time, Isabella thought she was struggling with everyone else's criticism, only to discover that her own critical mind was more abusive than any outside voice would ever be.

Upon further discovery, we started to understand how the pain that was controlling Isabella's choices belonged to a deprived little girl. This little girl who was in pain had been calling the shots, and she had equated all the junk food at Grandma's house and the free- dom to eat as much of it as she wanted with love itself. By letting her misled inner child control what she ate, Isabella was sacrificing control of her health, or lack thereof.

We set boundaries for this hurt little girl inside her as Isabella practiced saying, "You do not know how to parent me and were never meant to. That is not your role. I need to be the parent and let you know that too much sugar and junk food is not good for us. I need to let you express your needs and desires through feeling your emotions and understanding them for what they are: a cry for love and affection. I can find other joyful, healthy ways of addressing your hurt feelings. I need you to know that I am taking charge and taking care of all of me, which includes you."

This did it! Isabella started asking herself, "Am I really hungry? Do I truly want a potato chip?" The foggy pain continued to lift as Isabella's health improved dramatically. Then one day, like a last kick to the shins, Isabella's pain laid it out.

She had removed all junk food from the house and had gone several weeks eating in a way that was enjoyable to her and good for her body. Then stress crept back in. We were approaching Isabella's birthday, and the idea of not having a butter-cream birthday cake instigated a short-lived binge. Without wasting valuable time and energy punishing or shaming Isabella for her return to old patterns, we progressed to develop the thought, "I cannot possibly give up sugar because that is what is taking care of me. Don't make me let go of the only thing that loves and accepts me!"

Isabella started listening to herself, not all the chatter behind the craving, without judgment and criticism. She realized that shopping was one of her issues too. Whatever she could reach for, run to, or obsess over that could replace her real feelings was what she wanted. It had nothing to do with the cake or the new purse and everything to do with loving herself.

What Isabella needed more than anything was a healthy dose of self-love. Since the fog had started to lift, she could clearly recognize her overwhelming feelings of fear, anxiety, and resentment for what they actually were: the longings of a lonely and formerly lost little girl who needed to feel loved, like she had some purpose in the world.

Isabella understood that she needed to hold young Isabella close and tell her how precious, safe, and cared for she was. Isabella's Convergence Healing could not begin until she assumed some responsibility, chose not to feel sorry for herself, and set out to make a change. She not only had to teach herself to eat healthier, she had to unearth her core issues buried beneath the food.

As the pain of the self-abuse that was controlling Isabella's life lifted, she declared, "All I want to do is what is best for me and serves my health. No more eating out of the dumpster of self-sacrifice to ghostly memories."

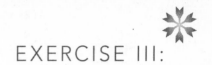

EXERCISE III:

JUST THE FACTS

If you are honest about reality, you cannot stay hidden in the fog. I have found that we get pulled deeper and deeper into the hazy comfort of the fog when we lose sight of the facts about our pain.

So here is a great exercise for you.

Write down, as well as you can, the facts around your pain. First write down the drama side that is comfortable in being the victim. This will probably be very easy. Then write down the factual side. Be sure to remove adjectives: Just the facts, please! Here is the fact checklist of my own story, to use as an example.

JUST THE FACTS: PAIN WITHOUT ADJECTIVES
The Facts of Peter's Pain:

Pain Story	*Facts*
1. I was in a terrible, fiery crash.	I died when my bike was pushed into a semitruck.
2. I met a messenger from heaven who rejected me.	He sent me back.
3. My body was badly, irreversibly injured.	I was in physical pain.
4. I was shamed and unloved.	I was depressed.
5. They did this to me.	I take responsibility.

Pain Story	Facts
6. My pain is my worst enemy.	I name my pain and make it my friend.
7. I am so sick and tired of living this way.	I embrace my pain and welcome what it has to teach me.

When you can understand the facts of your life, then you can do something about it. But if you keep living in the drama of the story, you will never be free and able to step out of the fog and into the freedom and spaciousness of true healing and health.

CHAPTER FOUR

Open the
Convergent Mind

Healing may not be so much about getting better, as about letting go of everything that isn't you—all of the expectations, all of the beliefs—and becoming who you are.

—Rachel Naomi Remen

The human mind is the greatest source of healing available to us. Not only that, it is absolutely free and is with us all the time. Instead of celebrating and using it as the great healing tool that it is, we have let our minds become (oh, irony!) the greatest single source of human pain and suffering known to mankind. That is because we, especially Westerners, are lax about taking care of our minds. We tend to let them run amok, preferring to give our thoughts free rein to create and reinforce harmful, destructive, and very entrenched patterns that keep us chained to our pain, and we stay very limited in our ability to live as authentically and freely as possible. The irony is incredible in our culture of healing in the West. We value freedom above all, and have built our country on its very DNA, but then so many of us have become trapped in thinking that there is really only one way to heal (allopathic medicine) and that healing is purely a physical problem that is treated through physical means.

We tend to have very little or no skill in approaching the mind with gentleness, curiosity, or, most important, love. Instead, we tend to approach our own minds with a sense of futility or resignation, even suspicion and dread, believing that our negative patterns of thought are intractable or worse. Yet there is no scientific or spiritual reason to believe that the mind is the enemy. On the contrary, there are countless studies that show how life-altering and healing cultivating and building healthy mind habits can be. We are fortunate to live in a time of great curiosity and scientific research on how the mind works. Part of the understanding of the human mind that is emerging is how miraculously flexible and self-correcting the mind can be, thanks to the lifelong regeneration of neurons and the great plasticity of the human brain.

We live in a time where there are many very effective non-invasive techniques we can turn to in order to free our minds from paralyzing ruminations, calm the inevitable reverberations of early trauma, and find our way to the sense of peacefulness that our human hearts so long for. These practices include meditation, neuro-feedback, cognitive behavioral therapy, hypnosis (of course), and others. There are many modalities one can engage in to soften and release the mind, to open and expand the mind. Once we become friendly with our own thoughts and our own judgments toward our habits of mind, only then can we find release and relief. Learning how to skillfully engage the mind is at the heart of Convergence Healing.

Now the principle universally laid down by all mental
healers, in whatever various terms they may explain it,
is that the basis of all healing is a change in belief.

—THOMAS TROWARD

We tend to approach our thinking in a passive way, believing
that if we spend any time examining our thoughts, we will become
even more insufferable and even more victimized by our thinking.
This can and does happen when we give our pain the power to dic-
tate the story of who we are. We are taught to believe that whatever
it is our mind tells us is the truth rather than viewing it for what it
really is, which is . . . just a thought.

Just a thought. Sit with that concept for a moment (or two).
What if you decided that every lousy thing you have ever told yourself is . . . just a thought? What if you knew that you could simply let
those thoughts come and go, or even better, that you could actually
change those thoughts and feel a hell of a lot better about yourself?
What if you believed that you could reprogram your thoughts so
that you felt less pain?

If I had realized that the miserable internal monologue that I
had lived with for so many years was not the gospel according to
the universe but rather a series of bad mental habits I had become
attached to after my accident, I would have reclaimed my life much
sooner.

It is not easy giving up that which we believe makes us who we
are. I believed that I was no more than the sum total of my accident.
I became completely blinded to the truth that my accident was just

something that happened to me. I actually became my accident, in body, mind, and soul, because I believed the thought that told me I was the cause of everything that ailed me. This was not true. My accident was not me. It could be me if I learned to reframe it and let it be a source of good in my life. What if, instead of continuing to feel victimized by that event, I really did start to believe that my accident was something that happened *for* me instead of something that happened *to* me?

This subtle shift in thinking cracked the healing universe wide open for me. Once I was able to make the tiniest bit of space for the possibility that there was some good in what had happened, I began to open and free my mind. I often tell my clients that I am grateful for the accident that killed me. If it was not for that experience, I would not be here with them.

THE DIFFERENCE BETWEEN TURNING IN AND TUNING IN

When our pain calls out to us, it is usually loud, anguished, and superdramatic: "Help! This is an emergency!" We respond to this over-the-top warning that something is amiss by turning all our attention to the site of our pain. This is a natural, even primitive response, as it is the brain telling us that on some level our life is on the line and we need to stop! We need to stop so that we can attend to the pain.

We get into trouble when, instead of just acknowledging our pain, we tumble headlong into it (like a swan diving into the abyss) without any guidance and forget that there is light and air and unlimited possibility above us. We hold our breath. We can no longer hear (especially reason). Our thinking freezes. We stop taking decisive steps. We become utterly consumed by our pain. Diving into your pain is good. Blindly being consumed by it with no lifeline secured to a knowing of peace or conscious stability is not.

This is the great turning point of our lives: we either heed pain's call and befriend it, taking in the message it brings, taming it with love, or . . . we ignore it, and it continues to wield its power over us from the shadows, getting worse, until it controls us.

We need to acknowledge our pain, see it for what it is, name it, and be honest about it, in order to release it.

While we must take responsibility for the pain we feel, we have to watch out that we do not become obsessed with it. Or consumed by it.

Turning too far inward for some can even be fatal. Think of all the brilliant, beautiful people who have become so overwhelmed by their pain that we have lost them to suicide. I myself certainly know the deep, bleak despair that can come with chronic pain; it is no wonder so many of us medicate ourselves with easy-to-come-by narcotics, or pharmaceuticals, or alcohol, or food, or sex. I mean, who wants to feel pain?

Convergence Healing asks you to communicate with your pain. As I've found out through this process, the sooner you embrace it, the sooner you'll be able to let your pain go and find your healing. But only by facing, naming, communicating with, and forgiving your pain can you heal. To wallow in it is often our natural instinct, but only because we don't have a plan to heal it, which is what I'm hoping this book creates for you.

Turning outward or externalizing our pain can be just as damaging as turning ourselves inside out when we have been injured. Often we look to others to fix or cure us because the pain we are in has rattled our sense of self-confidence, our sense of self-trust.

This is when we run the risk of becoming hooked on blaming others for our situation (if the driver of that car had only been more careful!) or turning to others to find out how to get better instead of trusting our own good judgment (I should have listened to my intuition and gotten a second opinion). Instead, we have this need to invite the input of others (Western medical doctors, therapists, holistic healers), and we give over to them all our power. "You're the healer/doctor. Heal me!"

The trick is to learn how to tune in to the gifts of others and then use what is helpful to you so that you stay in a position of personal power with your pain. When you do this, you let pain become a source of guidance and strength, a teacher in the way a good nutritionist or a dogged personal trainer can be. You stay in the position of decision maker. The pain will guide you, but you are the one who calls the shots. When you honor your pain and work to alleviate it in the ways that are most appropriate, the healing will radiate into other parts of your life.

Think of healing like a row of lined-up dominoes. When you get all the information you need (each piece set up in alignment before the last), you can take decisive positive actions, and the dominoes will fall as they are meant to, bringing immense relief and a sense of strength and wellness into all areas of your life.

SQUEEZE, PLEASE

Here is a great exercise to show you how when we grip down on something—a thought, a painful injury, a sense of injustice, or even our view of ourselves *as victims*—it can become impossible to see beyond that point of focus. So take a hand, put it out in front of you, and then make a fist. Now squeeze that fist as hard as you can. Focus on putting all your energy into squeezing your hand. While you are doing that, please keep reading.

Keep squeezing.

I could write anything here, anything at all, such as the alphabet or the lyrics to a favorite song or my mother's recipe for lasagna, and I bet you would not remember any of it if you were really trying to squeeze your closed fist as hard as you possibly could. When we become so set on controlling everything about ourselves, including other people's opinions, it is hard for us to realize that the world around us not only continues to spin but *it is passing us by*.

Yet, that is what so many of us do. We respond to pain by causing more pain. It is a vicious cycle: the more frustrating things become, the more we try to control them. There is no conscious living when we are trying to force life in this way.

How we exert control can be tricky and hard to identify. We've all got to cop to our control issues or we won't be able to break free of them.

I meet a lot of world-class people pleasers in my practice. But instead of thinking that this is how the person is wired, I've observed that these people pleasers actually use this "pleasing" to control everyone around them. Each and every one of them has a bad case of "like me–itis." I see this with clients who have a severe fear of public speaking: they simply cannot let go of their need to control how others perceive them long enough to speak up and let others decide for themselves. I see it in my clients who have emotional issues around food: if they are consumed with either bingeing, purging, or undereating, they will not have to attend to the realities of their relationships. The same can be said for those who have OCD or even issues like insomnia: whatever behavior serves to distract you from actively engaging in your life (like squeezing your hand into a painful, tight fist, for example) is something that can often be traced back to a fear of losing control over how others see us, which opens us up to truly being known (by oneself and by others).

The convergent mind is a mind that is willing to release control and move into a place of ever-expanding awareness and freedom. It is a mind that is willing to trust, to let go, to breathe, and to be.

Oh, yeah. Keep squeezing.

Is your hand starting to hurt? If so, why don't you open it, flex your fingers, and take a deep breath? While the numbness subsides and you feel the flow of letting go, I will tell you about another client.

BILLY

I met Billy when he was between jobs and failing miserably in all his interviews. He was oozing desperation, and his fear even made me sweat a bit. I had to take a step back, breathe deeply, and remind myself not to engage in my people-pleasing habit of taking on his stress.

Billy wore thick glasses that caused his eyes to appear a bit distorted, and so he had trouble meeting someone's gaze. This was particularly true when he was introduced to someone for the first time, especially someone he perceived to be more powerful than he, such as a potential employer.

Billy had worn eyeglasses ever since he was a small child, and he remembers well-meaning adults bending down over him and saying things like "Is he blind?" as though he were deaf and unable to speak. Actually, his glasses corrected his vision to near perfect, but the way they distorted his eyes made him, he believed, look "off." Since he believed this, he had adopted the unconscious habit of looking away whenever someone stepped close and made direct eye contact with him.

By looking away (which was a kind of "flinch" response), Billy telegraphed to people one of several things. Either (1) he was put off by them, or (2) he wasn't paying attention to them, or (3) he was not happy to be in that person's presence. Though on paper he was the perfect candidate for the job, he could not close the deal because he could not connect at that one key point of human contact and meet the gaze of any of his prospective employers.

I suggested to Billy that perhaps he was trying too hard to control how others might react to his gaze. I asked him if he had any particular memories of someone reacting badly to his appearance, and he told me about an awful instance of being teased and taunted when he was a child.

We talked about how working so hard to control the reactions of others almost always backfires. It is exhausting and the cost is usually higher than we can afford to pay. That is because the most important job we will ever have is to be our authentic selves in the world, and the way we do that is to meet the world head-on, without shame, to the best of our ability.

I told Billy I was jealous that he got to wear such cool, hip eyeglass frames, and he shared with me that his lazy eye would sometimes drift at odd times, which would inevitably make some people smile. There it was! The silver lining! Billy's relaxed and unexpected gaze could actually put people at ease. Plus, he was killing it in the style department with his fantastic frames.

Maybe, I suggested, trying to control who got to look into his eyes and who did not was not the best strategy for conquering the anxiety he had always felt about his appearance.

I asked Billy if we could end our session facing each other in a relaxed way, looking into each other's eyes, but only as long as it felt comfortable to him. Then, when he broke the gaze, we would both close our eyes and do a brief breathing meditation together. When we finished our session, we shook hands and then, spontaneously, we hugged.

Billy called me two weeks later to tell me he had landed a great job. He went into an interview knowing that his instinct would be to flinch and look away, and so, instead, he closed his eyes, took a deep breath, and then opened them, and he held the gaze of the person he was meeting with.

Billy's experience of opening—it might be our hand, our eyes, our hearts, our minds—was revelatory. He realized, as we all do when we begin to actively heal ourselves, that each small step he took to take care of himself with honor and integrity brought him to a new level of calm, a new level of peace.

He found that, as his mind opened, his heart began to heal.

BEING OPEN TO BEING WELL

This profound, very conscious opening of the mind is similar to what Buddha calls "surrender" and Esther Hicks, who channels an entity known as Abraham, calls flowing "downstream." It is what I think of as making the decision to be the river and not the rock.

When we surrender, we finally stop fighting. It does not mean giving up. When we stop fighting for our rightful place in the world, we allow life to open to us. When we take this first step, the step of letting go, we allow ourselves to become part of the natural flow of things.

The convergent mind is a mind that accepts reality for what it is and takes action from a place of expanded, big-picture awareness. It is a mind that has greater emotional flexibility and cultivates a heart that can "roll with the punches." When we are open to a true convergence with the universe, we move into a state of flow and we no longer get stuck on one particular problem. There is a power in being able to look at the facts of the life you are living as opposed to the judgments and opinions you or others might make about that life. When you become open, you are no longer prisoner to your pain or your fear, especially the brutal pain that judgment brings.

I encourage you to go ahead and give yourself the permission to free up your mind so that you can put the energy you used to pour into resistance and control toward your own deep healing.

NINA

On her seventh birthday, Nina's parents woke her up earlier than usual. Nina remembers feeling confused but excited as everyone in the family escorted her outside in their pajamas. There in the early-morning light, sitting in the driveway right next to her father's silver Buick, was a brand-new Barbie doll behind the wheel of Barbie's very own yellow-and-pink Winnebago. Nina was both happy and surprised.

The youngest of five sisters, Nina's relationship with dolls was perfectly normal until her older sisters figured out that, because she loved her dolls so much, they could use them to tease little Nina. The older sisters would pull the heads off her favorite dolls and chase Nina all around the house with her headless dolls in order to scare her. The older sisters would laugh and lock their baby sister in a closet with just her dolls' heads. She told me that she would just cower behind the locked door, sobbing her eyes out while she also squeezed them shut, so she wouldn't have to see her beheaded dolls. By the time she was ten, Nina's trauma had evolved into full-blown pediophobia, or a morbid fear of dolls. Every doll she had ever had either had to be thrown out or locked away.

During our first session together, Nina and I discussed her pediophobia. Did she truly suffer from a fear of dolls or could it be something else that had frightened her?

Nina revealed that after she became so fearful of dolls, her older sisters began protecting her. "Oh, we can't have dolls around anymore because Nina will freak out." It became a family thing. Every family decision was made so that Nina would not be traumatized, and this included making sure that no TV shows or movies featuring dolls were seen, no trips to stores with large toy sections were made with Nina, etc. It became so bad that Nina's younger nieces and nephews had to hide their dolls if Nina was coming over.

Nina's phobia was controlling not only herself but also her family and close friends. As the youngest member of her family, she had very little opportunity to assert herself, and the development of this phobia became an unconscious way for Nina to fight back against her sisters, who now felt terribly guilty for the fun they had had at her expense. But for many, many years, they were still paying for their bullying. Nina's fear held everyone in her family hostage.

Nina came to see me at the age of twenty-two because at that time she wanted to attend beauty school. All the work of hair styling and makeup application was done on lifelike doll heads. Nina had tried everything she could to desensitize herself to her long-held phobia. She had been trying to get past it for several years but had not been able to. She would enroll in beauty school and then drop out before the semester began. This time she wanted to see it through.

I asked Nina what it might feel like if she were to really stand up for herself. Since she had never done that before, I had her imagine, specifically, what it might feel like to call out her sisters on their bullying and stand up to them directly. She was controlling them indirectly, but she feared confrontation with them, which was her avoidance of her pain.

Even just my suggesting this felt overwhelming to Nina, so I suggested to her that she write four letters, one to each of her older sisters, telling them exactly how she'd felt when she was a child and they had tormented her. I told her to write each letter without judgment and to know that her letters would never be shown to her sisters. Basically, I was asking her to say everything to them that she would not normally say. I gave her permission to be as mean as they had been to her and to unload on them through the letters. She could swear, rage, and express every thought or feeling that she had shoved down around this issue of being tormented by her siblings.

I taught Nina how to put herself into a trancelike state and urged her to use this state of consciousness and write down every horrible thing that came to mind. Her instructions were to write for four days in a row for twenty minutes straight through.

The first day was tough for her emotionally, but the words flew out of her and the pages multiplied. Nina later told me that each night, after her writing session, she had incredible dreams of flying. When she had finished the fourth letter, she told me that she could no longer call up the deep charge she always felt when she revisited the abuse. She told me she felt like the pain of being abused had become ghosts that actually flew out of her body when she wrote about them.

On the fifth day, I asked Nina to write a letter from the future. I asked her to write from the future to her present-day self and to tell Nina how beautiful it felt to live without fear and that she could now have dolls in her life again, if she wanted to.

When Nina came in again, we did a burn ceremony and every letter was released into smoke. Ceremonial work like this can be really powerful when it comes to releasing traumas and pent-up energies. And it is really easy!

To start off the ceremony, take a moment to acknowledge what you are releasing. Say it out loud. For example, with Nina we said, "I release and uncreate the pain and separation I feel around my sisters and the fear of dolls." Place the letters in the fire as you recognize their power actually being uncreated and transformed into ashes. Finally, after the letters are completely burned, sit in gratitude and reflect on who you are without this pain.

Three simple steps: Acknowledge the pain, recognize it being uncreated, and give thanks as you visualize, imagine, and think about what life is like without the pain.

Six months later, Nina was beginning her second session at beauty school and she told me she couldn't be happier. Plus, she was still flying in her dreams.

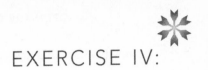

EXERCISE IV:

A VOW TO OPEN

A vow is simply an agreement, a promise that is traditionally shared between two people. It is a commitment to live a certain way. There are vows of celibacy, vows of fidelity, and even contractual vows that define a responsibility. This exercise is about you making a commitment to yourself to having an open mind and heart. It is to be made between you and your highest self, your happiest potential. I challenge you to take this vow and to make the promise to yourself to love and to cherish, to honor and to recognize, to listen and to open the space you need and deserve to be able to heal.

I, _____, with the universe as my witness, promise to love myself, all parts of me, absolutely and unconditionally.

I am willing to release the pain of control and to let my mind, body, and spirit move into a place of expanded openness, awareness, and creativity.

I agree to give voice to all parts of myself, and to love those parts with grace and ease, and especially to approach them with an open mind and heart whenever they are hurt. I promise to be kind, patient, and forgiving. I promise to do the work necessary to create a life of love and release.

I promise to understand every day and in every way the truth of my perfection. I recognize that I am an integral part of the universe, worthy of love, and that the truth of me is a gift that is to be shared.

I vow to share this love through the things I do and the words I speak.

I promise to do the work necessary to allow my healing to be revealed in the world and to love through the pain of growth, through the difficulty of change.

I promise to remain open to the processes of learning, growing, and revealing.

I welcome the challenge of being me with open-ended love.

I LOVE YOU.

_____   _____

(signed)   (date)

CHAPTER FIVE

Dissolve into the Present

You have to remember one life, one death—this one!
To enter fully the day, the hour, the moment whether
it appears as life or death, whether we catch it on the
in-breath or out-breath, requires only a moment, this
moment. And along with it all the mindfulness we can
muster, and each stage of our ongoing birth, and the
confident joy of our inherent luminosity.

—Stephen Levine

Now that you have made the vow to yourself to open your mind
and heart to the possibility of healing, it is time to work on releasing yourself from the shackles of your past and to relax your focus
on the future. It is time to step into this present moment, which is
the point in time where Convergence Healing occurs.

STOP!
READING!

Did those words startle you? I hope so, because if they did, it means you were truly absorbed in reading this book. You are likely a bit annoyed with me, because when we are actively engaged in an activity like reading, we are truly immersed in the present. I know how much I love sinking into a delicious book and losing myself into the "zone" of reading, where time as I know it dissolves and I am just . . . present with what is in front of me.

I am sure you know the feeling: you are utterly caught up in a task you love, be it cooking, or gardening, or making love, and something startles you. It is as though you are being called back to reality from a place of blissful, protected, sacred time. Once we are snapped back into the present in this way, our minds (and hearts) usually start racing.

So. You are here now. With me speaking directly to you. How do you feel? Are you annoyed with me for interrupting your reading? Are you curious about where this conversation is going? Have you become aware that you are thirsty? Hungry? Need to use the bathroom? Without me even posing these questions, your mind has begun an automatic querying process. If you pay attention to it, you will see that your conscious mind begins scanning for some kind of connection because it becomes anxious if it does not have something to grasp.

The mind is constantly trying to tether us to something concrete, or legitimate, or meaningful to say or believe. But what if you simply decided not to listen to what your mind was telling you? What if you decided to just let the questions that arise—and the inevitable dozens of micro-questions the big questions prompt— sail on by? What if you decided to just let your mind be?

Letting our minds "just be" is what living in the present moment is all about. By gently, kindly, and lovingly refusing to engage with our critical mind, we allow ourselves to sink into something that will nourish us (in this immediate example, it is reading what I hope is a soothing, inspiring book) and envelop us and allow us to become one with our experience.

This kind of peacefulness is what dissolving into the present is all about, but it is a state that few of us know how to achieve because so few of us have been taught how to cultivate it. Being at peace is something we all desperately need; it is the only state of mind we can be in if we want to experience true healing. Thankfully, we live in a time when more and more of us are engaging in practices that help us, in the words of the great Ram Dass, to "be here now." These practices include yoga, guided meditation, hypnosis (which empowers one to relax the mind), chanting, walking, singing, drum circles; there are as many ways to loosen our attachment to the distractions of the critical mind as there are flavors of pain. Pain, as we all know, is the ultimate distraction.

I knew I was on the right healing path when I began to feel more alive in the moment, more crisp and present and clear, more available to life. When I became comfortable owning and naming my pain, time itself seemed to relax for me, and I no longer felt as fearful about the future or as anxious about the past. Peace began to creep into my life for the first time, and I found myself waking to face the day with a growing sense of delight and curiosity. I began to realize that today was enough. I no longer had to tax my mind by trying to create a painful bridge between the traumas of my early life with the unknown of my future. It felt like I had been given permission by the universe to stop being so hypervigilant with my thinking and to just let it go and be. Just for this one moment.

Finally, I had learned to just accept my mind for what it was—a garden of thoughts that I could either let run wild with weeds (harmful thoughts) or gently cultivate with soul-satisfying nourishment (peace of mind). Gaining this understanding was a complete game changer for me. I finally began to understand that what happened to me was not who I was, that the events of my life did not make the man. What mattered was how I *responded* to the things that happened. I could either grasp the pain and continue to hobble through my life, or I could rise and walk in peace. I knew, once I got a glimpse of how spacious and powerful a moment could be, that I very much wanted to walk the path of inner peace and to enjoy a mind free of fear and filled with love and kindness.

———

We must cultivate our [inner] garden.

—FRANÇOIS-MARIE AROUET,

a.k.a. VOLTAIRE, CANDIDE

———

The human mind is a funny thing. We all have this perception that we are unique and that our thoughts are unique, yet every person on this planet has both a critical mind and a vast, untapped peaceful mind. I tend to think of the unobserved critical mind as the evil gardener, the trespasser who sneaks into the vast acreage of our minds and tears up all the beautiful flowers and fruits and instead plants aggressive, toxic weeds. This evil thought planter wants us to get tangled up in doubt, fear, and judgment. This "gardener" thrives on making you anxious, or in pain, or afraid of life. The more weeds he sows, the more painful our lives become.

Be careful not to punish this gardener. He is only doing what he knows. If tearing things up is how he knows to behave, then that is exactly what he is going to do. The challenge is to not beat him up like he beats us up. Instead, teach him a different way of being. He too needs to be loved.

So how do we get rid of those mental weeds? We begin by taking note of them, by identifying them.

Again, it is all about tuning in. You may tune in and catch your internal critic while, for example, you are engaged in your daily commute to work. Though you could, almost literally, make this drive in your sleep, you will note, if you pay a bit of attention, that your internal critic is busy backseat driving from the moment you take the driver's seat ("Buckle up!") to the moment you pull into your parking spot at work ("I wish the car in the spot next to me was not crossing the line"). We think we are actually being quiet at times like this, but our minds are racing at a hundred miles per hour, nagging us with so much judgment and criticism and hyper-vigilance that we can, literally, be overwhelmed—by our own minds!

A curious thing happens when you actually put your full focus on that mysterious voice in your head. If you tune in to that voice, it will quiet down. It will actually stop talking. Whenever we look at what the evil gardener of our mind is planting, we offer ourselves a moment of vitally important internal breath-taking. When you stop and quiet that voice, that internal critic, you become aware of the vast, open spaciousness of your mind, and you begin to realize that you can consciously choose to plant healthier, more loving thoughts there. This is when healing begins to happen.

Here is an easy visualization you can do whenever you find yourself still and seated (but not while you are busy, such as when you're driving a car):

Take a seat and plant your feet firmly on the floor. Close your eyes and take three deep, easy, relaxing breaths. Now think of your mind as a garden. What do you see? Is your mind bright, vibrant, and filled with your favorite plants and flowers? Or is it choking with weeds? Is there actually litter—old tin cans, barbed wire, empty plastic water bottles—in your mind's garden? What kinds of animals live there? Rabbits and sweet songbirds? Or snakes and spiders?

While you are visualizing your garden, allow yourself to relandscape it. If you would like, imagine yourself in a pair of well-worn Wellies and soft canvas gloves, coming through with a watering can, a weed whacker, or a wheelbarrow full of blooming flowers. Allow yourself to move freely around this garden, with purpose and delight. Once you feel satisfied that your garden is as verdant and fragrant and peaceful as possible, take a mental step back and just take it all in. Breathe in the scents of fresh grass, blooming flowers, abundant fruit trees—whatever you see that nourishes you, heart and soul. Let the sunshine of your inner garden warm you. Let the fresh, healing breezes of your open mind wash over you. When you open your eyes, you will be refreshed and renewed.

CLEARING YOUR MIND

My mind was killing me! Truly! I had been gathering evidence about how the doctors were right, how I was going to be in pain for the rest of my life, and how there was nothing I could do about it other than take drugs and have more surgery. And even then those things wouldn't help. I could not think about anything else, and the constant chatter of pain was driving me crazy. There was a part of me that knew it did not have to be this way, but that healthier, more reasonable voice was small and insignificant compared to the abusive chorus of pain that was repeating over and over again in my head.

I began to imagine what my life would be like if I had to use a cane, a wheelchair, or, worse, be dependent on others to help me. The fear this kind of projection instilled in me was nearly paralyzing.

Luckily, I had enough understanding about how the subconscious mind works. I remembered an old adage that says, "What you pay attention to grows" and finally . . . I got it. I understood that the more I focused on the pain as pain and not as a messenger in disguise, the more hopeless I felt about ever feeling better.

When I realized this I made a decision. I decided that I would do whatever it took to change my abusive and wounded thinking. I had no idea how, but instead of focusing on fighting the pain and resisting the thoughts it was trying to deliver, I decided I would turn toward them.

So I started to practice loving the parts of me that were hurting, and I began to ask them what they needed from me. My pain told me that what I wanted and needed to do was to find peace. What I needed to do was meditate.

I tried several different flavors of meditation practices, including Transcendental Meditation, or TM, and mindful meditation. For me, a combination of these two became my own unique style of meditation. I experienced a sense of mental relief that really kick-started my healing process. Since then, there has been a tremendous amount of scientific research into the healing benefits of meditation, and researchers at the Center for Functionally Integrative Neuroscience at Aarhus University, in Denmark, discovered that meditation even helps our brains to continue to grow. Scientists from the Department of Psychiatry and Behavioral Sciences at Emory University, in Atlanta, discovered that regular meditation can stave off the negative mental aspects of aging, such as memory loss and decline in cognitive functioning. Meditation produces "positive" neurochemicals like nitric oxide, which stimulate blood flow, which in turn relaxes the heart and can positively affect 1,561 of our genes. In fact, there are no negative effects to meditating!

There are so many ways to meditate that my best advice is to find the practice that works best for you. Some people prefer to sit with a group and follow the meditation prompts of a master or teacher who leads the group into a state of focused relaxation. (This is not dissimilar to what happens with a hypnotherapist and a client or a group.) Other people prefer to meditate to tapes or even YouTube videos. Others prefer to meditate alone as a form of prayer. The whole purpose of meditation is to silence those nagging voices in your mind, even if it's just for a moment or two. The benefits are vast and difficult to measure, but the resulting feelings of serenity and calm are undeniable.

There are also two styles of how you can approach meditation. One is a focused meditation. This is when you practice focusing your thoughts on a single thing, be it a movement, a sound, or an object like a candle's flame. The next form of meditation is called mindfulness. The practice of mindfulness is to actually notice everything and let it go. The metaphor that worked for me to understand this better was to visualize, imagine, and think about sitting on the side of the road and watching the cars go by. There goes a red car, there goes a blue car . . . Just notice and let go.

When you jump into the car, that is when you have been hijacked by that thought, opinion, or judgment about that car. Simply recognize when you have jumped in and get out. No posture, no mudra, no special carpet or beads required.

When I work with my clients I actually take them through both these styles of meditation. We start with a focused meditation, move to mindfulness, and then dive into a hypnotic trance. Our minds can be wounded with worry and be healed through meditation.

During my work, I've learned that the brain cannot hold a negative thought at the same time as a positive thought, and so I encourage my clients to adopt a simple mantra that can consciously remind them that this fact is so. My own personal favorite is "Faith, not fear," and when I repeat this phrase to myself, I am consciously encouraging my mind to release fear and replace it with faith. It works every time.

When we make a commitment to ourselves to actively strive to cultivate our minds with healthy, nonjudgmental, and life-affirming thoughts, we begin to release ourselves from the grip of pain. Life begins to take on new qualities of "worthwhile-ness" and we allow ourselves to step out of a state of being "unworthy" into a state of being valued and loved. We are no longer prisoners to the wicked, critical gardener we all have lurking around the edges of our minds. Instead, we have begun to train a new gardener, a presence that is kindly, wise, and gentle. This gardener understands that patience truly is a virtue, one that we need to bring into our lives in abundance.

CULTIVATING PATIENCE

I think it is safe to say that I have not always been the most patient person. When I died, I was furious with the messenger I met on the other side who insisted that I had to return to earth and figure out how to live my life differently. I was so angry and resentful by this perceived "rejection" that I spent the next two decades of my life steeped in bitterness, regret, and all-encompassing pain. Of course, I finally got it that I could not simply wait for my pain to diminish on its own: I had to take the steps to actively heal myself first by engaging it as a teacher. I had to take charge of my own health, to take ownership of my broken, battered life.

In order to do this, I had to learn to be patient. I had to learn to let the lessons of my life reveal themselves to me at their own pace and in their own time—instead of being constantly pissed off that I was not somehow "better" right that very minute.

Even acknowledging that I needed to learn patience was enough to bring me to my knees. I needed this. I needed to get humble around my shortcomings in order to release them.

For so long, I believed that I was ugly and unlovable, and these negative core beliefs kept me stuck in a horrible cycle of really un-healthy, even abusive relationships. Without even being aware of it, I became a magnet for partners who were financially insolvent, deeply wounded emotionally, addicted to alcohol—you name it. If someone came into my relationship radar with a psychic garden that was more choked and polluted than my own, then I was all in! I became a master of rescuing wounded boys and killing myself trying to change them and turn them into men. Though they might look different on the outside, the men I kept choosing were emo-tionally stunted and committed to a dependent approach to life. As one of my close friends would point out, I would choose a different shirt but the same man. I refused to acknowledge this pattern.

Instead, I positioned myself as the victim time and time again. ("It's not me, it's him!" was my mantra.) My reward for this kind of arrogant, codependent behavior? I would be left exhausted and brokenhearted. This pattern of engaging in one bad relationship after another went on for years, until I finally decided to just stop. To finally let myself be alone.

Until I picked up with another guy whom I allowed to fill my garden with all kinds of weedy, allergy-producing crap.

This is where kindness and patience needed to come in. I had to forgive myself for clinging to this unhealthy pattern. I finally began to understand that beating myself up for making bad boyfriend choices was the linchpin of this unhealthy cycle. Once I acknowledged my unhealthy impulses with love and compassion, I was finally able to step out of this awful habit and to approach relationships from a slightly less toxic point of view.

This is where the garden metaphor becomes so crucially important. A garden is a living, growing thing and it needs our consistent care. Weeds are inevitable. So is drought or deluge or infestation. Our job, as the cultivators of our own minds, is to stick with it. To return to the garden (our tangled minds) over and over and over again.

On some days, we may do a little weeding. We may trim the hedges with a rather dainty pair of clippers.

But there are times in our lives—say, after we suffer a major setback, trauma, breakup, or injury—when we have the opportunity to go in and clear-cut the whole thing.

These moments, when our minds are ripped open and we have the opportunity to make radical changes to our belief systems by releasing unhealthy patterns of thought, are rare gifts from the universe. As a healer, I have come to realize just how rare they are, and when a client comes to me, open and vulnerable and honestly ready to make real change, this is where the Convergence Healing magic happens.

BRENDA

This was one of those hypnotherapy sessions that started with me thinking, "How am I going to help this person?" I confess, there have been many times that I have had this thought. Each time I say a little prayer, hand it over to God, and lean into my trust of the Convergence Healing process. It works every time.

I did not know most of her story (and still do not), as I never focus too much on the why or how, not wanting to get lost in all the details of a client's past. I really want to keep assisting clients in the present moment. All I knew at the beginning of our appointment was that Brenda had been suffering a lot of aftershocks due to an extremely traumatic event in her past.

At some point in the not-too-recent past, Brenda had been one of those women whom we hear about in the news who was trafficked and held as a sex slave. Again, I do not know the entire story, but she was under someone else's power. There was a lot of manipulation, pain, highly abusive treatment, that type of thing. It may have even been for quite some time, as long as a year or two.

My relationship with Brenda was not about the past. It was about who she was in the present and my being of assistance in helping her create the life she wanted in the now.

Again, I do not have clients go into their stories. These are traumatic experiences and we are not trying to reactivate them. I only get enough information to begin the steps of Convergence Healing. And while we are going down that path, I remain focused on the moment and always try to maintain a sense of awareness around what was the past and what is now.

During my first session with Brenda, something happened

that I had only heard about but never witnessed. Brenda literally collapsed. She was sitting on the couch and we had just started the meditative process that I use to get people into a trance. I had not gotten her fully under when there appeared to be a surrender experience for Brenda. She simply tipped over on the couch and remained in this position for the majority of our session.

Her eyelids were fluttering. It was as if she was experiencing a sense of complete powerlessness, frozen in the trauma of what she had experienced. This must have been one of the ways in which Brenda had learned to survive her captivity, to completely shut down and go into a numbed-out state.

As we kneaded our way into this physical experience, working toward actually knowing what the experience felt like, I needed Brenda to recognize what her body was experiencing at that moment. Not what was in her head, not the details of her story as she tells it, not the deep vat of emotion connected to it, but the physical experience of that trauma in Brenda's body at that present moment. Until we address the feelings of our trauma, it does not matter what we think of it nor what work we do around it emotionally.

While Brenda was in this trancelike state, I appealed to her conscious mind, letting her know that in this quiet moment she was safe. I asked Brenda if she agreed, and she responded yes by nodding her head. We began the process of teaching these painfully traumatic memories to find their way back to their proper place in history. Brenda had to understand that these events were not actually happening in the present, even if her feelings of numbing out to survive felt the same, then and now. The pain still had that much of a hold on her.

Why was I trying to make her go there? I was not. Remember, trauma gets stuck in the body, like a ghost that does not know its time has passed. It does not matter how much you think about it, you are still experiencing it. It is as if it is still happening and has not been processed and released. And Brenda, although she was coping with the memory, was still managing a survival-mode filter of numbing out when she felt confronted or threatened—whether it was by her loving boyfriend or even her beautiful child. Confrontation, no matter where it came from, was always responded to by shutting down and numbing out. This was Brenda's fog and she was done living in fear of it.

I remember movies and TV from when I was a kid. There would be the Vietnam-veteran dad now living in Idaho who would be barbecuing with his family in the sunny backyard, and *boom!* Some loud noise would trigger a reaction and he would be down on the ground back in Vietnam. He could smell the jungle, see the enemy.

In his consciousness, he was not in Idaho. He was in that traumatic experience that happened a long time ago that he kept pushing back into the recesses, but it still surfaced. The moment this trauma was triggered, it took over.

You may have a conversation with yourself that begins, "Why am I having these thoughts and feelings? I do not want them." You may try to shove them down. This will not work. I see this a lot with my clients struggling with addiction.

They can be sitting at the bar, ordering their tenth drink, and their conscious mind says, "You really don't need that." At the same time their emotional self screams, "Please don't drink that." The survival experience is always going to bully the conscious and emotional brain into submission. Someone struggling with addiction may drink as a way to fight off the pain of the world, he may drink to flee and run away from the world, he may drink to freeze and numb out, or he may drink as a way to try and hide.

What those feelings need is to be felt and released. We may have done a lot of emotional work and cognitive work around the trauma, but the actual physical experience is most likely still stuck in the body.

Even though her head did not want to go there and her heart screamed that it was beyond this, the experience of the trafficking was still stuck inside Brenda. When she walked down the street, someone moving in a shadow would trigger this trauma and her body would begin to panic. She was in a constant state of suppression, trying to shove the fearful thoughts away and simply walk along freely. Her body would become flush, amped up, her heart pumping wildly.

It was very powerful to get Brenda into that experience of just acknowledging what it was like in her body, where she could hold space for it and be present with it. After our session she said that this concept and the actual doing of it was liberating. She realized how tired she was of having to always shove down this numbing response and struggle to stay present.

What is that stuff still inside you, held in captivity? What is it like in your body? Using all your senses to know it, what does it feel like? From being patient with yourself to feel through it, from this place of witnessing and not reactivating, you will move forward. What does it taste like, what does it look like? Sit with it, allow it to be present. For those reluctant to revisit horrifying traumas, remember that if you still feel emotionally charged when the incident is brought up, then it is still there and active within you.

Trauma is always hanging out. As Brenda peeled away the layers, I continued to ask her to recognize with the conscious mind that this experience of being trafficked was not happening in the present moment, even though she was still feeling it. This separation may seem obvious, yet it is crucial.

I asked Brenda, "Is there anything in this room right now that is causing this survival reaction to kick in?" She said no. I asked her again if she realized that she was safe in the moment with me. She said yes. I told her that the experience she was feeling was not really happening at that moment. She said she understood that when I asked. I explained it was an old traumatic memory that we were recognizing, a memory that needed to find its way back in history to where it belonged. In doing this, she could retrieve that piece of her soul that had been left behind, still suffering and holding her hostage in the present through the pain that remained orphaned in her past.

This usually affords the client a healthy distance from the effects of the trauma: I am feeling this and it is okay because this is a safe place to feel it. Know it deeply.

It is so important to be able to discern the actual separation between what you are feeling and what is actually happening. Go beyond just a concept of the feeling, get physical, go gritty. The only way we know things is through our senses, so use them.

Recognizing your pain allows it to be processed. Once you know it and recognize it, it gives you something to work with. All this stuff was going on in Brenda's body, but she knew it was still not really happening in that moment. She could now identify what she was feeling and remind herself that the physical experience was a thing of the past.

This distinction qualified her to begin working on the trauma while reducing the confusing emotions connected with it. And with this, we brought in the mantra "already done" as a way to teach the parts of her holding on to the memory to let go and shake loose the stuck memory. "Already done" is a powerful phrase taught to me by my chi gong master. I asked Brenda to put that phrase and the vibration of it into the part of her that was numb.

Brenda began to clearly identify what her pain felt like and could recognize it. She discovered that the numbing experience actually lived in her chest (lungs and heart). It was hot, heavy, cold, and closed at the same time as it was dark, black, and stabbing.

The more we recognized it, the more the pain let go. Instead of shoving it down, we had created an opening for it to be processed. Brenda now put the mantra "Already done. . . . Already done . . ." into her heart. She even brought in some drums to build a rhythm, and the sounds began to shake loose the tightness.

We continued teaching the pain itself and her experience of it to find their way back in history by having Brenda visualize a comforting coolness that soothed the hot inflammation and then a warmth that melted the cold. She found herself on a tropical beach, feeling the warm sun and the cool waters. To the darkness we brought in a beautiful glittery bright pink light, and to the sharpness we invited an experience of velvety smoothness to come in. As she did this, all her fears kept coming to the surface.

One after another they would show themselves, and she would lovingly notice them and let them go. Her focus was on the color, temperature, sound, and feeling of teaching this old memory to find its way back in history. The fears were just things that had attached to the trauma, and as it vibrated away from her into her past, the fears too dissolved. I asked Brenda if the need to numb out in order to survive was still there, and with a big smile on her face she said no.

Next, I asked Brenda to go back in time to the first incident she felt she needed to numb out in order to survive. She quickly responded and said she was nine years old. Apparently, numbing out was something she had done even before the trafficking. We found the nine-year-old version of her and I asked her to whisper into her heart, because they shared the same heart, the words "I love you." As she did, a tear slid across her face. Brenda sat up and we continued the session from this new position.

Remember, Brenda had been sitting collapsed with her head down on the couch almost from the moment we started. I told her that we had gone back in time to help this little girl heal and to remove her from any danger. Then I asked her to let the little girl know that she was loved. Brenda said, "I'm already hugging her." With that, we brought both of them back to the present and I asked Brenda what she needed to take this healing to an even deeper level.

She had learned that she needed to dance again. Once, Brenda had been a very social person. Now she was not, and that needed to change. As a playful, creative soul, she had to allow herself to be seen and not be afraid. From her younger self, Brenda spoke: "If I am seen and recognized, I can do stuff to learn to trust the world and myself again. I can build my strengths. That cannot happen when I am home alone." Brenda's younger self was very clear and immediate on the things that she needed in order to heal.

Mentally, she wanted a hug. For Brenda this was less of a body/physical request and more of a mind request, because it was a way for her mind to learn how to trust again and discern who was safe and who was not. She wanted to stop listening to everyone else's opinion about life and the way she lived it.

Physically, she needed a shoulder massage and long, luxurious baths; to get her hair done and to stop looking in the mirror and being cruel. Brenda used to constantly tell herself that she was ugly. Her little girl was very clear that she wanted none of that. "Get new clothes," she told Brenda.

Spiritually, Brenda's younger self set a very solid boundary that it was not okay to lie to herself or anyone else anymore. "I will not tell myself harmful stories about who I am anymore. I refuse to listen to anyone who tells me I am not 'enough.'" The younger self demanded that she stand up and be heard.

This is an extreme example of almost instantaneous "clarity," but while most of us will not experience a trauma this harrowing, we will experience spontaneous healings like this by following the steps of Convergence Healing. Some of us will heal more slowly, over time, like I did, and that is okay. We will walk a more ordinary, human, and divine path where we will cultivate patience and practice dissolving into the present so that the inner workings of our minds are revealed to us. To achieve this state, we must learn to invite our minds to engage in meditation, which is a fancy word for resting in peaceful silence.

I love knowing that meditation became a "thing" tens of thousands of years ago, when ancient people lapsed into a peaceful state while staring into the flames of their campfires. I like to imagine these ancestors, tired and dirty from a day spent hunting and gathering, seated shoulder to shoulder, all eyes tracking the dancing flames. I can put myself there in a heartbeat, and I can feel the warmth of the fire on my face and hear the crackle of the wood burning, smell the smoke, while my mind dissolves into nothingness. Inevitably, just imagining this brings a smile to my face.

That is the feeling of true meditation. Peace. Ease. Belonging.

Finding the right style of meditation for you is superimportant. Someone who has an anxious mind probably is not going to have much success in attempting to engage in a silent meditation. When your mind is already having difficulty handling silence, giving it more silence can be maddening. It is a little like letting all the crazy chatter that anxious individuals experience loose in an empty hall: the echoes bouncing off the walls get louder and louder.

Remember, there are all kinds of meditative practices, from sitting with your legs crossed in silence to chanting mantras, listening to guided meditations, walking meditations, and mindfulness. I have developed an "active meditation" for my clients, which helps achieve this beautiful trancelike state. It is an easy exercise that can be used whenever needed or desired.

EXERCISE V:

CREATE A TRANCELIKE STATE

If you have ever taken a long road trip and found yourself on a flat, empty stretch of highway, there is a good chance that you have likely lapsed into a state of semi-awareness that state troopers like to call "long-distance drive trance." I know I have become so relaxed that, the next thing I know, I'm driving over the speed limit and have lost all track of time and space. I have even driven past the exit I was looking for and continued down the highway for miles. This is when you might get pulled over, and if you are asked, "Do you know how fast you were going?" by a state trooper, your honest answer will be no.

This phenomenon is the trancelike state I want you to learn to develop and harness—but not when you are driving or operating heavy equipment! This kind of meditation needs to be practiced in a place where you will not be disturbed, if possible. You may also practice this technique when you are on a plane, train, or in the middle of a crowded waiting room. I often tell clients that they'll know when they have mastered this technique when they are able to do it in the middle of Grand Central Terminal at rush hour. The only criterion is that you need to be left alone and free to be able to allow your thinking to tune inward.

I always stress that my way is simply an example. The more a client modifies the language used to induce a healthy trancelike state for themselves, the more effective and meaningful the experience will be.

STEP ONE: JUST NOTICE

Sit, get comfortable, and just notice. Focus your eyes on something in front of you. Name the thing and let it go. Notice your breath, your breathing. Look at something else. Name it and let it go. Notice your body. Just feel that you are here, now, in the present moment. Notice it all and then let it all go.

STEP TWO: BREATHE

Take a full, deep breath. Hold it and comfortably count to ten. As you release it, count from ten back down to one. Do this mindfully and with a relaxed, easy frame of mind three times. If your eyes want to close, great. If your shoulders drop, even better. When your mind quiets, you are there.

STEP THREE: DISSOLVING INTO THE PRESENT

Now that you are in a state of peace, I want you to count backward, from ten to one, and as you take in a deep breath, follow these steps:

10. Notice how relaxed you are becoming.
9. Let yourself enter the stillness of your mind.
8. Feel the calm wash over you.
7. Listen to the ocean of your breath.
6. Give yourself permission to become even calmer.
5. Notice how the energy of life is flowing through you.
4. Notice that stillness flows through you too.
3. Notice how open your heart feels.
2. Notice how peaceful your spirit feels.
1. Notice that you are free.

You have, however briefly, just utterly dissolved into the present.

Open your eyes. Welcome to a new world where peace replaces pain. You are now freer and more integrated into the gorgeous mystery of life than you were just a few short moments ago. This is the place where mind, body, and soul converge.

This is exactly where you want to be.

CHAPTER SIX

Love Inside Out

Find the love you seek, by first finding the love within yourself. Learn to rest in that place within you that is your true home.

—Sri Sri Ravi Shankar

For far too long, pain ruled my life. I let the pain that had begun in my broken body and fragile, easily disappointed young spirit define every aspect of who I was. I do not know if it was because I was so young and impressionable, but I let myself become pain's slave, a true victim. I believed that I was helpless in the face of my pain—that pain was my judge, jury, and jailer.

I actually used to believe (and had settled into the fact) that I would be held captive by my pain for the rest of my life. This helplessness translated into my not only feeling but acting as if I was already defeated. I was resigned to a life of frustration, cozy inside my crestfallen attitude of "Things will never change."

Are you stuck in a downward spiral of disappointment? Is "It will never work" always your first thought whenever a new opportunity to find relief reveals itself? Are skepticism and doubt your go-to emotions around healing your pain?

Because of these debilitating beliefs, I had to learn this truth the hard way: when you live in a prison of pain, everything is colored by it. Hope is dulled, joy is fleeting. Enjoying love and true intimacy feels impossible. There seems to be nothing that is not influenced by the pain.

For so many years, my pain was etched on my face, lodged in my bones, choking my voice, and polluting my thoughts. Like an oil slick, it darkened every aspect of my being. It even had a taste, a dirty, cold metallic taste, like a quarter I had picked up off the street and decided to suck on.

I consider myself one of the lucky ones, because despite being in chronic physical pain most of my life I somehow managed to escape my painful prison long enough to remember that there is love in the world. Although I still experience pain regularly, I no longer allow it to limit me or be a deterrent to my happiness.

At first, the presence of a bit of tenderness toward your pain may startle you. It startled me. I felt it with the therapists and healers I visited, kind people who genuinely cared about my being well again.

Most profoundly, I remembered love when I finally experienced a bit of compassion for myself. At that moment, it dawned on me that the gate to the prison I had been cowering in had been unlocked and open all along. I had been so busy hiding my face in shame that I never looked up to see that all I had to do was walk through the gate. All I had to do was put one foot in front of the other and carry myself away from the pain and toward love.

Of course, isn't there always a catch? I could do this only if I learned how to truly love myself. One of the ways I did this was to make amends. When you become willing to apologize to yourself for some wrongdoing, the ego becomes threatened. It will want to distract you from revealing a perceived vulnerability. Do it anyway. In the long run this will actually strengthen the ego and help it transform into a mighty lover as compared to a sniveling fighter. To make amends to yourself is to apologize for your ignorant past wrongs and ill treatment.

I apologized to myself for continuing the shame that was thrust upon me by what we know as a conservative society and the organized religion that would denounce me due to my being born gay. I made amends for beating myself up and for punishing myself for being who I am. I made amends to my spirit for the abuse I had inflicted upon it, to my body for the shame I gave it, and to my mind for not respecting and caring for it better.

I did this through writing love letters to these parts of me. It felt silly, frightening, and invigorating, but, most of all, liberating. Yes, I get that it sounds kooky, but the process of making amends with myself opened up my heart to love again.

This is the true quest that is at the heart and soul of Convergence Healing: each of us must learn to love ourselves mind, body, and spirit, wholeheartedly and unconditionally, if we are truly going to become whole and authentic.

If you have spent your life savaging yourself, hating yourself, and caving in to the inevitable pain that life brings each of us, this "learning to love yourself" will probably be the most difficult skill you will attain in your lifetime. But learn it you must if you truly want to be free of pain.

Pain of mind is worse than pain of body.

—LATIN PROVERB

Love is the key to releasing you from the prison of your pain. The love I am talking about is radical acceptance of the self. This means accepting not only your flaws, limitations, and weaknesses but accepting your pain.

I am not talking about simply acknowledging pain as a symptom. For example, I suffered from chronic sciatica ever since the accident almost thirty years ago. Only recently have I been able to heal this pain, after finally uncovering some layers of pain from long ago that were causing the "symptom" of sciatica. I am talking about understanding the root cause of your pain, which usually means getting really clear on your feelings and getting honest about all your fears, hang-ups, biases, and other limiting or debilitating habits of mind that keep you beholden to pain.

It is only when we learn to love and honor the source of our pain—be it issues brought on by early abandonment, neglect, or a lifelong sense of shame, resentment, regret, or physical injuries—that we can truly release it and find lasting relief in whatever form that will be: emotional, physical, or spiritual.

Let me present a prime example of what I am talking about: a friend whom for purposes of anonymity we will call Samuel.

SAMUEL

Samuel and I are polar opposites. I am all about moderation and treading lightly, whether in regard to politics, religion, and especially health. I always advocate for a noninvasive or nonpharmaceutical approach to healing, even when it comes to pain.

Samuel, on the other hand, believes in the power of the prescription and the almighty word of anyone who has the letters *M* and *D* after his or her name.

Samuel has suffered terrible neck pain from an old sports injury for as long as I have known him. I once suggested that he might benefit from practicing some meditation, even some gentle yoga, but he just laughed at me. He has a very stressful job in finance and finds all my "Eastern woo-woo meets modern boo-boo" activities to be, well . . . quaint, shall we say?

About a year ago, Samuel heard about a cutting-edge surgical procedure that spinal surgeons had been using with success, and so he sought out a local doctor who would perform the surgery on him. I remember when he called me to tell me that he was "psyched" to have the procedure so that his neck troubles would be over for good.

The surgery went smoothly and Samuel emerged from the long, painful postsurgical physical therapy feeling confident and well. He seemed to get earnest satisfaction out of telling me that his neck never felt better and that he never once had to light a candle or chant a prayer.

That is, until he called me about six months after his surgery and told me that he had awoken with not just neck pain but also a massive headache. He had put in an emergency call to his surgeon, who put him on the schedule for the next day. After a thorough physical exam and then an ultrasound of his neck, the doctor discovered that Samuel had a bulging disk right at the site of the surgery. Samuel's doctor's best option? More surgery.

I had to bite my tongue from saying "I told you so," and instead I let Samuel begin the dialogue about why this might have happened to him. As it turned out, Samuel was feeling so cocky postsurgically that he had double-downed on his work, and he found himself constantly craning his neck to talk to clients on his cell phone at all hours of the day and night. When he would finally put his phone down (he has clients all over the world in many different time zones) he would be so depleted and stressed-out that he had to have a few drinks before going to bed. Then he would get a terrible, short sleep and get up and do it all over again. His neck was a mess, but he had also put on about fifteen pounds. The overworking and stress resulted in his wife being on the verge of leaving him, and he never saw his kids.

Perhaps, I gently offered, it was his work that was causing him so much pain and not simply his old sports injury.

I had offered up this opinion several times before, but this time Samuel heard me. He finally admitted that he could not be the "superstar" finance guy his father insisted he be. Samuel needed to take a step back, if not for his health, then for the sake of keeping his family intact.

Samuel realized that it was not more surgery that he required. What he needed to do was reassess how he was living his life and begin asking himself important questions about purpose, passion, and his basic wants and needs.

In short, Samuel had to turn his very "other"-centric focus in on himself and begin to nurture his own heart and soul. Only then would his body truly begin to heal.

After we had this conversation, a funny thing happened in my relationship with Samuel. We became closer. I discovered that I liked him more and more as he started to shed the macho "master of the universe" finance jock persona he had been perpetuating with such stubbornness over the years. I realized that under the tough-guy exterior was a pretty thoughtful and caring man, the true Samuel I had been drawn to in the first place.

He even came in to see me for a session of Convergence Healing. During that brief hour, Samuel released a lot of pent-up shame around feeling "not good enough" in the world, especially in relation to his father. He was stunned to find that, after just a brief encounter with his true feelings, the pain in his neck subsided considerably and he was able to sleep more soundly than he had in years.

FINDING THE COURAGE TO LOVE

I believe there is nothing more heroic than mustering the courage and strength to identify the true source of one's pain and then release it by healing it with love.

But this process takes fortitude, bravery, and a willingness to give up the idea of being "perfect" and opting instead for becoming whole, integrated, and at peace. Pain is an integral part of life, whether it is the pain of childbirth, the pain of grief and loss, the pain of genuine remorse, or the pain of falling out of love; pain is part and parcel of the human experience. Pain is a primal experience that transcends the physical and influences our soul and spirit more than anything else except love.

Pain gives our lives contour and meaning, and without it we would never get to experience the deep compassion we need in order to become truly intimate with ourselves and with others. Pain takes perfect out of the picture and allows us to just be, without judgment, without expectation.

But what happens when we are afraid of letting go of our pain? What if we find ourselves clinging to our pain, to the strange anti-comfort our pain has afforded us for so long?

Resistance is a normal part of growth. Think of the first time you did something that challenged your sense of your own limitations. It may have been something you now take for granted, like jumping off a diving board into a pool.

Close your eyes and imagine yourself at four or five, when you probably weighed less than fifty pounds. Remember how steep the steps on that metal ladder were, and how cold they felt under your small feet. Remember how it felt when you finally stepped onto the diving board, which was a foam-green plank covered with sandy bumps, like a giant emery board. And remember, finally, how it felt to get to the end of the diving board and curl your toes around the edge.

Nothing ever seemed so high before. Nothing ever seemed that dangerous. But there you were. You may have looked over your shoulder, your heart sinking as you realized that going back and trying to get off the board would be more dangerous than stepping off into thin air. But for that moment . . .

If you are like me, your stomach is doing a flip just imagining this now.

Somehow or other, most of us mustered the courage to take a breath and fling ourselves off that diving board, and before we hit the water, we knew everything about our lives had changed.

That is because we had pushed through that wall of resistance; we had quieted our fear just long enough to allow ourselves to take a giant leap of faith into the great unknown.

Splash!

When we came up for air, we were different people. We had pushed ourselves beyond what we knew we were capable of, and we found that, in an instant, we had grown.

The trick now, especially when we are in pain, is to keep ourselves supple enough of spirit to push past the resistance we will meet when we need to release all the emotions and thoughts we have locked up within us by that pain.

I help my clients break through this wall of resistance by encouraging them to befriend their pain. Really own it.

One of the ways I do this is to urge them to adopt the following mantra:

"My pain is perfect. It is exactly what I need."

This phrase may strike you as silly—and it should, because it is so counterintuitive and unexpected that it is pretty damn funny.

But it is also profoundly true. There is no greater teacher, no wiser sage, and no better guide to self-knowledge and self-acceptance than our pain. In this way, our pain truly is perfect.

We can add to the mantra like this:

"My pain is perfect."
"It wants me to feel _____."
"It wants me to know _____."
"It is here to alert me to a part of myself that needs my attention and care."
"It wants me to acknowledge and name something that has been hidden for too long."
"When I name it, I may release it."
"My pain wants me to grow."
"My pain wants me to heal."
"My pain wants me to be free."
"My pain wants me to be whole."
"My pain wants me to love and be loved."

By juxtaposing the word "pain" with these nourishing words, we resist the urge to demonize it, and so we can bring it in closer to our hearts and our understanding.

Our pain is not the enemy. It is simply a messenger, a signal that we need to attend to a part of ourselves that we may be ignoring or abusing. It is like a bell that is calling us to prayer, a phenomenon, a sensation that is meant to bring us to attention and to awareness. It is a guide, a teacher, a sacred mentor, if we let it be. In this way, nothing is more perfect than pain.

Befriending your pain is a revolutionary act. In a society that wants us to numb out, hide out, and silence our pain at all costs, naming and owning your pain can be downright subversive, which means that there can be an element of risk to it. It may confuse your loved ones and alienate others. It may even elicit a hostile response. (For example: "I can deal with you when you are down-and-out, but how dare you rise and shine?") Being brave enough to say "I am in pain because of this (fill in the blank)" means you are serious about healing yourself. When you make this kind of bold declaration of self-care, you have firmly stepped onto the path of Convergence Healing.

GRATITUDE BEGETS LOVE

When I was just beginning to heal myself, as I mentioned, I spent a lot of time in Al-Anon, where I learned the power of gratitude and the importance of making amends. Making amends is not the same as apologizing for something we have done that hurts another person, although apologizing sincerely when we have done wrong is also something I learned there. Making amends means acknowledging the cost of your actions and making a vow to try, to the best of your ability, to do things differently in the future. I came to realize that the person I most needed to make amends with was myself, and so, along with practicing gratitude on a daily basis, I also practiced forgiving myself and others and making amends so that I was clearing the way for new, healthier behaviors.

Several years later, I came across the beautiful ancient Hawaiian healing practice of ho'oponopono, which is a type of mental cleansing, a form of emotional and moral rebalancing that brings harmony to one's spirit and heals the wounded relationships the practitioner may have with others. There are four phrases used in ho'oponopono to cleanse the spirit and to reconnect you with your truest essence:

I love you.
I am sorry.
Please forgive me.
Thank you.

You can say these phrases in any order (though the sequence above is the traditional order), and you can practice this when you are alone. But it is very important to say these phrases out loud and with sincere, heartfelt conviction and repeat them until you find yourself transitioning into a state of true relaxation and calm.

At the heart of ho'oponopono healing is the belief that everything we experience is something we have created within the confines of our minds, so it is our responsibility to lovingly cleanse our minds in order to keep from lapsing into a state of mental passivity or victimhood.

I love the four phrases of ho'oponopono and I visualize them as beautiful, luminous small seashells that I wear on a soft string as a precious necklace. When I feel stressed-out or flustered or simply overwhelmed, I reach for these pearls of wisdom and recite them, and I immediately feel fortified, clear, and balanced.

IF YOUR PAIN IS LITERALLY KILLING YOU—WHAT THEN?

In our culture, we tend to fight real medical calamities with a "warfare" mentality. How often do we hear that someone we love is "battling" cancer? Or "beating" some disease or another?

In Convergence Healing, we trust that love and acceptance are more potent healers than aggression.

I am not saying that one should forego traditional medical treatments. In fact, with severe, life-threatening illness, it would be irresponsible to not avail oneself of the wonders of modern medicine. But I do feel that any form of Western or allopathic medical therapy can be augmented and improved by the addition of a Convergence Healing practice.

When a person is in the throes of a life-threatening illness or disease, it is easy to lose the vital, healing grounding in one's innermost essence. Convergence Healing practices steer a sufferer back into the safe haven of his most essential, authentic self, and this is the place where miraculous healing happens. It is here, in the deepest well of our one, true heart, that we can shift our consciousness and find our way to a better space, even if it's not on this physical plane. I know this firsthand, and I have spent the better part of my life trying to reconnect with myself in the heavenly place of knowing I experienced in an instant so many years ago.

JAMES

As a therapist, I sometimes work with clients who "get under my skin." James qualifies for this distinction. An awesome seventy-five-year-old man, James came to see me in the late phase of stage IV cancer.

At first, James kept saying that he was not ready to die. All his actions, thoughts, and words were about leaving a legacy, however, about cleaning up his financial situation and healing relationships before he passed.

We started to talk and it came up that James had married his best friend in high school. He spent fifty years in a relationship that he recognized as unfulfilling even before getting married. Neither one of them was ever really "in love" with the other. Throughout his marriage, James had multiple affairs. Once, he even walked away from an extramarital soul mate in order to return to his first role as dutiful husband. James felt deep anger and resentment about staying married and regret for not following his true love.

James and I focused on making amends to himself for not following his heart's dreams. He was able to recognize all the times that the universe had offered him an out from the painful life he had committed to and say, "I love you" to the pain. The tears began to flow, and as we went through the process, James's pain melted away.

He began to say "I love you" to those whom he had felt wronged by. He thanked everything from his children to the tumors for the lessons that they had taught him. He made amends and apologized to his wife for staying in their relationship and empowering her guilt, which kept him right by her side.

Here was James, at seventy-five years of age and dying of cancer, asking forgiveness from his children for not being the father they needed. We did many exercises over the following weeks that helped us discover a deeper sense of love inside James. Our time together was fascinating!

As the cancer spread and his body became weaker and weaker, James's spirit only became healthier, more vital, and stronger. It was like witnessing his shedding of "this mortal coil."

The last time I saw James was in home hospice care. He asked me to come and talk with him.

He was beaming when I saw him. The light of his soul was shining so brilliantly that it lit up the room. As we sat together, we laughed, we prayed, and we talked about love, gratitude, and the power of forgiveness. With his relationships healed on so many profound levels, James was truly at peace. James passed away the very next morning. I was told by his wife (who no longer saw me as a threat) that with his last breath there was a smile on James's face.

What is so beautiful and serendipitous about this practice is that it covers everything that ails the practitioner. This can mean a long-standing issue of physical pain, distress over a troubled relationship, or frustration caused by lousy traffic conditions. It can even be a reaction to news of an environmental catastrophe halfway across the globe or a military conflict between countries that are in no way connected directly to the sufferer. You can begin to loosen your pain's grip without having to go into the details of it; you can simply ask for its forgiveness, thank it for bringing you to a new state of awareness, and allow true love to flow between you and the discomfort.

Before long, you will be awash in peace.

RESPOND TO YOUR PAIN WITH LOVE

In Western medicine, we are told that pain is actually a cluster of hot, overstimulated nerve endings—something that is, quite literally, under our skin.

But your pain, when you turn toward it and become curious about it, can take on very tangible qualities, such as a color, a texture, a fragrance, or a taste.

When you become truly curious about your pain, in the way that you are when you meet a potential new lover and are aroused and intrigued and eager for information, your pain will surprise you with how specifically it can manifest.

JANA

Jana came to me after she had tried to quit smoking several times. She had stopped for a few months, so we knew that it was possible for her to stop, but she eventually picked it back up again. She was quite upset over her painful predicament, as the smoking was completely out of alignment with how she saw herself as a person.

Jana is a vegan, a holistic health advocate, and a yoga teacher. Obviously her need to stop smoking was paramount, as she viewed herself as a "traitor" or a fraud of sorts. How could she guide people to live a healthy lifestyle when she herself was doing something that was the opposite of what she taught her students? As a coach, Jana was struggling, and her smoking had caused her to reach the level of a spiritual breakdown.

The first thing we needed to do was to get Jana "off the hook." The punishment and shame that she was heaping on herself only added to whatever anxiety was causing her to smoke in the first place.

Jana was caught in a loop. She saw herself as being better than the part of herself that was smoking, and yet she was still a smoker. This discrepancy between her two views of herself that could not merge created conflict, abusive feelings, and shame for Jana. This resulted in tension and anxiety in her body. The more she shamed herself, the more stressed she became. The more unmanageable the stress became and uncomfortable she felt, the more Jana reached for some outside source to help suppress her anxiety so that she could get on with her life.

As we worked together, our focus had to shift away from the smoking itself and onto the emotional experience that was causing Jana's need to smoke. First, we realized that Jana smoked only at home. From there, we dug a little deeper into the stressors she was experiencing at home.

Jana was in a parasitic relationship that she felt she could not end. Her boyfriend relied on her for everything, from money to his self-esteem. Jana's entire life was revolving around his needs.

We discussed the dynamics of this relationship and discovered an abusive pattern of self-denial that we were able to trace back to Jana's childhood. Jana had grown up in a home replete with addiction and undiagnosed mental health issues. As a child, she was not allowed to tend to her own needs. If she did, she was punished. Jana had learned to survive by suppressing her needs and putting the needs of others above her own. Sound familiar? Regrettably, it is a pretty common story.

As I mentioned, Jana earned her livelihood as a holistic health advocate and yoga instructor and was a pretty evolved person. She had just been living in a survival pattern of self-denial for decades, always too willing to do everything possible to make other people happy. Perhaps this fed her success at work, but not so much at home.

As we continued our sessions, keeping our focus on releasing Jana's addiction to cigarettes, we were able to set parameters that initiated her Convergence Healing process. On the mind level, Jana enrolled in a class on Buddhism so that she could study and occupy her mind with the principles of equanimity. On the physical level, we literally extended the time between cigarette puffs, drastically reducing her daily number of cigarettes. She also started to substitute carrot sticks as oral alternatives to smoking.

These were easy things for Jana to initiate, as they were already in alignment with the person she was. Establishing boundaries of where, when, and how much she could smoke was proving successful, but she was still having one to three cigarettes a day. Jana's goal was to quit smoking altogether, not simply cut back.

As we created some changes and the cigarettes began to lose their hold on her, we also jumped down into the trauma experience of having to put everyone else's feelings first. We discovered that her smoking was a way for Jana to say "Screw off" to those who had been her suppressors. It served a profound purpose of individualization for this little rebel girl asserting herself in a world where she felt very little governance over her own life.

We began a discourse with this rebel girl. Her name was Dawn, and was Dawn angry! Dawn felt ignored and abused and as if she did not matter. Dawn felt tightness around her heart, as if it were being strangled. There was a clamping-down feeling in her throat, a black heaviness in her chest. The smell of the cigarettes themselves, which she hated, suddenly appeared in the room, and the taste was like dirt.

Through Jana's ongoing conversations with Dawn, we asked what she needed in order to heal and quit smoking. Dawn replied that Jana needed to put herself first instead of last. I asked Jana to ask Dawn what this would look like in the world, and Dawn said, "I want to feel at rest! I need peace and calm!"

With this, Jana started to tear up. She knew exactly what Dawn needed her to do, but she had been putting it off. In our sessions, I would help guide Jana to a deep, calm, meditative state. At the beginning of the session there was always a craving to smoke, and whenever we adjusted her state of spirit (notice I did not say "state of mind"), Jana no longer had the craving.

Experiencing this peace gave Jana the wonderful surprise of knowing that she did not need to smoke to adjust her consciousness. Jana made the connection that if she practiced this state of being regularly, then the cigarettes would no longer be needed. Meditating was the answer Jana's spirit needed.

So Jana started to put herself first and did things that nurtured her. On the spirit level, we created a calendar that blocked out time throughout her busy day that was dedicated to just Jana. This was time for meditation and prayer and only that. As Dawn, the rebel girl hiding inside her, began to receive the attention she needed, Jana started to learn what it was like to love and nurture herself. The more her inner needs were met, the calmer Jana felt.

Adding to this, we started to teach the parts of Jana that were in pain what it was like to have a different experience. To the tight, strangling feeling around her heart we introduced a brilliant sunrise that allowed her heart to expand. To the tightening in her throat we brought in the rumbling vibrations of the sound "om." To teach the memory of the cigarette smoke we brought in the smell of mountain sage, and to the taste of dirt we brought in the knowing of cinnamon. The more she brought in the knowing of the smells, sounds, colors, etc., of her healing, the more calm she felt, and the less Jana felt the urge to turn to smoking for comfort. Success!

UNIQUE QUALITIES OF PAIN

The longer I work as a healer, the more certain I become that there are infinite variations in how pain is experienced or perceived. I think of pain as being like snowflakes: no two people experience pain in quite the same way.

There is no single way to heal pain either. The recipe for healing that you create using the Convergence Healing process is totally unique to you. There are no cookie-cutter, one-size-fits-all solutions here. Getting curious about your pain allows you to get a more nuanced and detailed visual, sensual, and mental awareness of the nature of your pain. I ask my clients to take note of these aspects of their pain:

> What color is it?
> What does it smell like?
> Does it have a climate around it? (Is it wet, cold, dry, hot?)
> Does it have texture? (Is it soft, slippery, hard, sharp?)
> Does it give off a sound? (Are there phrases it repeats?
>   Profanities? Noises? A soundtrack?)
> Does it have mass? (Is it heavy, light, dense?)

When you begin to think about the physical attributes of your pain, often it will actually take on a recognizable shape.

When your pain has taken on a physical form, it is time to ask if it has a name. My clients have surprised us both when they have told me that their pain was named Barnaby (a goat), Shelly (an octopus), and Mike (a black voice of doom). Often, pain does not have a name, and so I encourage my clients to give their pain a name.

Once you feel that you have located your pain outside you and it has taken on an identifiable physical presence in your mind's eye, and you have named it, then ask three essential questions of it. "Okay, pain . . ."

"What do you need to heal on a mental level?"
"What do you need to heal on a physical level?"
"What do you need to heal on a spiritual level?"

You may be surprised by the answers your pain provides.

EXERCISE VI:

LOVE LETTERS TO YOUR PAIN

One of the writing exercises I created for my clients is Love Letters to Your Pain. Writing is a very important tool for facilitating Convergence Healing, so make sure you allow yourself lots of time with a notebook and some fabulous pens or pencils. Once your pain is acknowledged and freed, it will want to communicate with you.

Every day, for four days, I want you to write a love letter to your pain. These letters should detail all the things you love about your pain. To do this, you simply take the most prominent features of your pain and you flip them on their heads. To elaborate, there was a client that I treated whom I will call Carrie.

CARRIE

Carrie suffered from chronic fatigue syndrome. For her, one of the worst symptoms of this illness was severe vertigo. Carrie became so debilitated by this that she was bedridden for days at a time.

Usually, Carrie never discussed her vertigo with anyone because it made her feel ashamed. She became like a powerless child again. Her mother even once accused her of filching the symptom from the classic Alfred Hitchcock film!

In her love letters to her pain, Carrie addressed her vertigo directly, saying that without it she would not have had such a keen appreciation for the days when she was upright. In another letter, she thanked her vertigo for making her bedridden so that she was able to study and complete her master's degree a semester early. In a third love letter, Carrie told her vertigo that she was very grateful for its visits but that it was now time to go. In the last, she continued to tell her vertigo that she loved it and even created a list of all the ways that she could continue to love it with gratitude for how it had served her.

Within a few days of writing these four love letters, Carrie's vertigo went into remission. She was able to leave her bed. Today, Carrie is living proof that the application of energetic love can heal.

Try writing to your pain the love letters it needs to receive, and allow the healing to begin.

CHAPTER SEVEN

Develop Deep Self-Trust

As soon as you trust yourself, you will know how to live.

—Johann Wolfgang von Goethe

Being brave enough to name our pain and to acknowledge it as a part of who we are takes a lot of trust. Trusting yourself, knowing you have the discernment and senses to make peace with your pain, is a skill that most of us are not taught.

One could say that a parent's most important job is to help a child develop a sense of confidence in his or her ability to engage in deep, meaningful self-care. But too often, our parents are grappling with their own limited relationships with trust. Unfortunately, those who are meant to guide us are not always on a tranquil, trusting path themselves.

Self-doubt and anxiety run in families, passed down from one generation to another, like the jewel-green eyes of a beloved great-great-grandfather. Negative family traits become entrenched and difficult to identify. We are told that we simply come from an anxious clan or that fretting is in our DNA. This may be true, but the innate ability to trust and to feel—especially the ability to trust ourselves—is also there in us, waiting to be discovered, developed, and celebrated.

Stepping into my own Convergence Healing not only lessened my pain, it gave my self-confidence a powerful boost. For the first time in many, many years, when I finally began my quest to heal, I experienced an awakening of internal strength and fortitude that I had no idea existed within me.

Taking action on behalf of my own well-being was the first step in awakening my ability to truly love and honor myself. Finding that I could trust myself to make healthy and positive choices changed everything for me.

When you trust yourself, you are no longer a victim of anyone or anything: trusting yourself means you have connected with your divine agency, your deepest life force. It means you are in touch with your vital essence as a unique, very valuable human being. But it can take awhile to get there.

One of the more hideous aspects of pain that often is not discussed is how dehumanizing it can be. When we are crippled by chronic pain, we believe we have become "less than whole" in the eyes of others, but in truth, we have become "less than whole" only in our own eyes. Pain, when it is allowed to run the show, becomes the ultimate bully and can strip us of our sense of integrity, our sense of competence, like nothing else.

But how can we expect to actively heal ourselves when we perceive ourselves to be weak, victimized, or incapable?

The truth is, we cannot. Without deep self-trust, pain wins. In order to heal, we must develop a loving, trusting relationship with ourselves first and foremost. This is a cornerstone of Convergence Healing.

Developing self-trust is a gradual trial-and-error proposition. You have to be willing to step out of your comfort zone and take new and different actions. After a while, the "different" actions will become your norm. This can be something as simple as saying no to an invitation from a friend when you have personal responsibilities that need to be addressed first, or it can be as profound as eschewing surgery in favor of trying a less invasive, perhaps more spiritually based form of healing first. It also means being absolutely forgiving of yourself when you take an action and realize it is not the right one for you. Developing true self-trust means learning to reset your positive intention and starting again.

Trust and forgiveness go hand in hand. We have to step out of black-and-white, right-or-wrong thinking and into the vast unknown of living authentically, which is a dimension beyond judgment and criticism. It is the place where we allow our true essence to emerge, where we allow our souls to rise, walk, and run.

For myself, transcending all my limiting beliefs and habits meant working hard to free myself from a fugue state I had been trapped in for years upon years. For so long, I was caught in a place that had me wedged between what I was told I *should* do and the hard wall of my inability to query myself lovingly and kindly. It was difficult for me to determine what it was my intuition, my wise internal guide, felt was the best course of action for me. It took a lot of effort for me to clear the debris of self-doubt and step purposefully into an empowered, self-trusting state of mind. It is a process I will continue to work on and refine my whole life long.

My professional work grants me great joy and a level of satisfaction that I have not known since I danced onstage, and possibly did not even know then. Working with others to discover and connect with their inner well of trust has given my life a sense of purpose that humbles and fulfills me.

In the years that it took me to begin to truly heal, I literally stumbled from one healing modality to another. Whenever I had enough money and someone suggested a healer that they had success with, I went to see the person. Some were just okay, but most of them were amazing. All of them offered me at least a small degree of healing that I would not have received if I had simply popped a pill and myopically hoped for the best. The interesting thing was that I would definitely get better, but the healing was always slow to take hold. My ability to absorb what I was being taught deepened as I opened myself to more options and new ways of thinking about my pain and what it meant to heal myself.

During that time, there was a lot of talk in the allopathic world about combination therapy, and it got me thinking. In Western medicine, the idea was to combine multiple drugs to combat a disease, so what if I combined multiple therapies to bring about a deeper sense of healing than what I was experiencing? I thought: Why not?

I had no idea how to decide which therapies I should put together. Then I started to look at friends who were struggling with weight loss. I saw that most of them were focused only on diet and exercise, but I knew their stories and there was almost always a wounded little girl or boy under the surface who felt unworthy and broken. That was when it hit me.

I started to actually apply the healing work that I was doing through a mind, body, and spirit approach. I had undeniable and obvious pain on every level of who I was. My knee and back were in unrelenting pain, my thoughts were constantly in turmoil, and my heart was clearly broken and suffering under the heavy shame I carried.

Indeed, I was my own best guinea pig, and so I tried various healing methods until I discovered those that worked best—for me.

When I began working with clients, I encountered the same resistance in them that I had had to overcome in myself, but once each client was able to embrace the idea that pain is a gift we should accept with gratitude and openheartedness, radical healing and personal transformation occurred. Once a client begins to name his pain, an open, active relationship with pain begins. Pain becomes the teacher, the teacher about how to choose living over shame, fear, and agony.

I began to watch my clients experience profound breakthroughs, and my trust in the evolving process of Convergence Healing grew.

I discovered that, by sharing my own story, I offered my trust to my clients, and they were able to make the leap of faith more readily. This sharing of my own trust deepened my connection with my clients.

There is that in you—Spirit—that is unconditioned regardless of what you have done to condition yourself.
—DR. RAYMOND CHARLES BARKER

For me, learning to trust in my abilities to help myself heal instinctively guided me toward seeking out my highest self. This seeking out of our higher self puts us in connection with the divine source of all life and healing. This is where the great energizing love that is at the heart of Convergence Healing resides. It is within each one of us, and our job is to seek it out and to strengthen our bond with something greater than ourselves.

I used to get angry with anyone who represented God or any institution of religion. I did not accept any higher power as part of my healing team, or any team. Being turned away from heaven after my accident felt like God did not want me. How wrong I was.

As I mentioned, I was brought up in a traditional Catholic household, but the way my family practiced its faith felt pretty rote and rule-based to me. After my deadly accident and otherworldly experience, I was so angry with the God of my upbringing that I rejected him wholesale. It never dawned on me that this was not necessarily God at all; this was a fictional person, a construct that I had been told to believe in, and I did my best (as the ever-dutiful, people-pleasing son that I was) to do so. But I had no native connection to this concept of God. It was not until I connected with the divine spirit within myself that I awoke to the awareness that God is not just one thing. God is radiant, energetic love, and that love is meant to be fully experienced by each of us uniquely and privately.

After my years in Al-Anon, I knew that I needed to connect with the source of my own wisdom, to identify with a higher power, but no one told me that I had to find that source of strength by tapping into my own inner strength first. Once I figured this out, I was able to connect the cosmic dots. Through practicing self-love and working to deepen my trust in my own higher power (my own innate wisdom), I would be able to connect with the universal higher power that actually informs every religion on earth, every healing practice, every thought, word, or gesture that stems from unconditional love.

Reconnecting with my inner wisdom reactivated my spirit and opened up my understanding of organized religions and beliefs so that I could harbor less judgment, less fear. I can sense, almost immediately, if someone is using religion either as a way of hiding out from the truth or as a way to punish oneself or others. When I focus on the love and goodness within the people I am working with, the energy of healing bypasses all limitations, skepticism, or biases present.

It is truly remarkable to watch the energetic healing love of Convergence Healing dissolve barriers of misunderstanding that keep us from being present with one another as we heal.

Convergence Healing put me in direct contact with my own higher power, and I felt, for the first time, less alone on this path of mine. Feeling supported by the loving, kind energies of the universe gives me more strength, more hope, more belief in my own abilities to heal.

Convergence Healing is about bringing all the good within us into alignment with the goodness that surrounds us. When we trust ourselves in this process, the universe responds in kind. Why not have all that healing power on our side?

After my accident and experience in that otherworldly, spinning tunnel of swirling white clouds, I came to believe that our spirit is our highest reality. What occurs to me in the physical world is, I believe, a manifestation of the state of my spirit. This does not mean that "bad" things do not happen to me. What it means is that, when bad things happen, I immediately check in with my spirit and ask it what it needs. Usually, there is a blessing in any challenge. A blessing that may not be initially apparent.

WHAT IS UP WITH CARS AND ME?

Recently, while I was writing this book, I was in another car accident and suffered a traumatic brain injury. At first, I was incredulous. How could this happen twice? Then I became angry. How could my luck be so bad? Shortly into my recovery from a bad concussion, I realized that perhaps sustaining a second injury to my brain was a way for the universe to direct my attention to my mind and to my physical brain. Maybe I had to really take the time to have my head checked out properly by some highly skilled Western doctors.

Everything seemed fine at first. Then I started having this headache centered behind my right eye. Eventually the ache turned into something that felt like a spike being driven through my head and I ended up in an emergency room. Writing and reading became more and more difficult, and there was dizziness, nausea, and a strange sensation like I could not open my eyes wide enough to focus, but somehow I continued to work with my coauthor and carry on with the writing of this book.

This recent car accident felt like a reliving of the previous one in which I had been slammed into that semitruck. Unfortunately, I have been in quite a few fender benders, but this one was different. It was as if there were residual things that had not been healed after the first accident, and this latest incident was giving me the opportunity to heal those things.

One of those unresolved issues was my anger. As a result of the concussion, I found myself feeling like that foggy-headed seventeen-year-old who could not think clearly and who felt lost trying to hobble through his last months of high school. The parallels were striking.

Again I was hit from behind. The impact was entirely unexpected, and since I did not see it coming, I could not react or prepare. Again I hurt my left knee. And again I hit my head.

This accident tapped into a deep well of unexpressed anger in me. I was plunged into the ancient sensation of having no control over my life. Here I was trying to finish writing a book, and I could not focus my eyes long enough to read a sentence, let alone sit at a computer and work.

I had to really lean on my writing partner, our editor, and my publisher, and trust that what we were all creating together was going to accurately represent the work I do, be well written, and inspire people suffering from all types of pain to heal—all while I was struggling with my own deep pain all over again. I had no choice but to make a leap of faith. I had to let go of my anger and trust. It worked, you see, as you're holding this book, and I was able to energetically love the old hurt that had lingered the furthest from my reach. And here we are now, on a journey of healing—together!

ALISON

Although I often guide my clients away from recounting the details of their life stories, Alison was different. She had been through something so unspeakably horrific that I knew, intuitively, that talking about her experience was crucial to launching her Convergence Healing.

Growing up with an abusive father, Alison had had a difficult childhood. She married an abusive man, and he left her during a bitterly cold winter, cutting off the gas so that she had to raise their children in a home with no heat. After that, Alison turned to a man for emotional support after her husband had left, only to be gang-raped by him and his beastly accomplices.

When I asked Alison what she wanted my help with, she replied that she needed to be able to trust people again. I understood, given what she'd been through, that this was what she'd think, but I sensed that there was something deeper she needed to address. So I asked her, with deep love in my heart, "What do you really need?"

Alison told me that at this point in her life she was afraid of being abused and taken advantage of by pretty much everyone she encountered. In order to keep herself and her children safe, she felt that she had to be alone and isolated. The only people she felt she could trust at all were her mother and uncle, and she was even beginning to doubt them—even though she understood that there was no practical reason for her not to trust them.

I took a risk and jumped right into the Convergence Healing process with her. With deep compassion and an emphasis on getting to the heart of the matter, I said, "Alison, I do not care how you were raised or that you were raped, abused, tortured, and betrayed. What I do care about is helping you figure out how you can move forward and find peace and happiness in your life again."

She was, of course, a little unsettled by this bold statement, but she understood that my intentions were good, and so we continued. Alison told me that she'd been attacked just six months before our session, but I knew that she'd been victimized long before that awful day. I understood, on a deep, intuitive level, that she had been putting herself in harm's way for a very long time, due to her believing that she was not a valuable human being.

I asked her when she had decided she wasn't worth protecting, when she had turned off her intuition. She told me that she felt it was at around age ten when she finally caved in to the belief that men (because of her abusive father) would only ever harm her.

We went back to that fateful August afternoon when Alison arrived at her boyfriend's house and walked into what she described as a "nightmare trap."

"You know, when I pulled up to his house, I realized that there were just so many cars there. Whose were they? He was usually home alone. It felt weird to me. I was getting a hit that something wasn't right, but I ignored that."

"You ignored your inner guide," I said quietly.

"I did!" Alison said, her eyes welling up. "I didn't listen to the warning!"

We talked about how the universe has a tendency to hit us harder and harder and harder until we get the message. It was horrible that Alison had to suffer this kind of attack before realizing that she needed to learn to put her own safety first and to trust that she could stop positioning herself within harm's reach of abusive men. It was time for Alison to start living her life for herself.

I pointed out that she was lucky. She had an inner guide that she could still hear—even if she had chosen, on that fateful day, not to listen to it. Her healing would entail her learning how to deeply listen to this voice and to act on its wisdom.

We started going through the Convergence Healing steps, and I could see Alison visibly relax. I asked her: "What if we talk to the little girl who stopped listening to Alison's truth? What if we asked her to join us right here, right now? What if we asked her what she needs to feel safe and cared for?"

Immediately, Alison said, "Oh, she wants to run." I asked if this meant that young Alison wanted to run away and hide. "Oh, no," she replied. "When I was a little girl and up until the rape, I loved to run. Running relaxes me and makes me feel strong all at once."

There it was! There was an action Alison could take that would make her feel more trusting of herself, more in tune with her deep well of inner strength. Alison promised me that her healing would begin with her going for a run. Even if it was just a brisk jog around the block—this would be the crucial first step.

What else could she do that would help her to feel safe? "I think I should probably take a self-defense class." What a great idea. "How does thinking about this make you feel? How does it make your younger self feel?" I asked. "She's jumping up and down right now," Alison said with a smile—the first I'd seen all day. I praised her for choosing activities that would shore up her physical health.

I asked her what she might do to help heal and soothe her spirit too. She told me that she'd always tried to find some quiet space to read and write when she was a girl, but her drunken father would invade any space she found. So we talked about her carving out some quiet reading time. We also discussed the possibility of her returning to church, which had once been a sanctuary to her.

Alison had a very strong, actionable Convergence Healing plan in hand. "Are you willing to do these things in order to create your health?" I asked. "Yes!" was her answer.

Before Alison left me, I shared with her a meditation, a prayer I developed for deepening one's sense of self-trust. I use it myself when my spirit turns toward despair and hopelessness rather than faith and healing. I've found that this prayer helps quiet the mind and taps directly into a very powerful, sacred energy source that we all have within us.

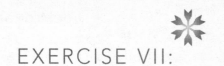

EXERCISE VII:

A PRAYER FOR SELF-TRUST

Find a quiet place to sit comfortably. Make sure that you don't have to use the bathroom, that you aren't thirsty, and that your phone is quieted. When you are seated, close your eyes and take in a deep, cleansing breath. Then ask the universe, or God, or spirit, or the divine goddess—or whatever source of loving, energetic healing you feel in harmony with—to light the path to wellness with your highest integrity, your deepest wisdom, and your most loving, authentic self.

RECOGNIZE

Recognize that you are an important, beloved part of the universe and that you are connected to all beings everywhere. In recognizing this fact, you affirm your connection to all the beauty and abundance in this world.

AFFIRM

Affirm your own value. The universe does not discriminate; we are all worthy of love, health, and peace in this lifetime. Remind yourself of this. Affirm your magnificent value as a human being and as part of the infinite cosmic family.

RELEASE

Release any resistance you have to feeling the energetic love the universe is bathing you in. Let go of any negative thoughts, opinions, or beliefs you hold about yourself. Release judgment and release the pain you have been in. Release it all and open yourself up to love.

ACKNOWLEDGE

Acknowledge that it is already done. With all your heart and every cell of your being, believe it when you say:

"I am whole and perfectly healthy."

"I am joyous, healthy, and free."

"The universe wants me to be free of pain."

PRACTICE GRATITUDE

To stay connected to your highest self, practice gratitude. Be grateful for this moment. The universe will take care of you if you pray for love, peace, and good health.

Say out loud:

"I am grateful that the universe loves me."

CHAPTER EIGHT

Integrate Trauma

The conflict between the will to deny horrible events and the will to proclaim them aloud is the central dialectic of psychological trauma. When the truth is fully recognized, survivors can begin their recovery.

—Judith Lewis Herman, MD

Nothing causes more pain and suffering than trauma. Trauma is an experience that is so overwhelming, either physically, spiritually, or emotionally, that it arrests our ability to feel safe in the world. We hear a lot about big traumatic events on the news, such as war or natural disasters like hurricanes and earthquakes. These traumatic events are loud, visual, and undeniable on a sensory level. But these traumas are, mercifully, relatively rare. What is more common and less easy to detect are the day-to-day traumas that we suffer, the slings and arrows of everyday life that may get lodged within us. Over time, these injuries, if unattended, remain open wounds that can begin to bleed and weep and hurt whenever we brush up against them.

These wounds leave us broken and afraid. And though they may be hidden from the rest of the world, they powerfully color our own perceptions and can keep us from finding our way to wholeness and wellness.

The vast majority of people who come to me for help are either knowingly or unknowingly suffering from the symptoms of unresolved trauma. Trauma is, I believe, the cause of much of the world's great pain. Trauma can destroy trust and crush a soul like no other force on earth.

Whether the roots of a client's trauma rest in the physical (like my car accident) or the psychological (warfare, rape) or the emotional (loss, betrayal), my Convergence Healing mission remains essentially steady and unchanged: to go within, understand how the pain is being held within you, name it, and allow it to tell you what it needs to heal.

Let's go back to the garden metaphor. Trauma is like a snake that lives in your garden. Most of the time it stays hidden, living away from your awareness. But if you inadvertently step too close to it, it may rear its head and frighten you. What if you were to discover, however, that this snake has no venom? What if you were to discover that this snake has no power to cause you further harm?

For my clients who suffer from PTSD or any of the myriad symptoms of unresolved trauma—which range from addictions to sleep and eating disorders to issues with emotional regulation and physical illness—the noninvasive, loving, and judgment-free practices of Convergence Healing can transform trauma and neutralize its negative effects.

The American Psychological Association defines "trauma" as an overwhelming emotional response to an injurious event. Deriving its meaning from the Greek word for "wound," trauma has had holistic practitioners agreeing for thousands of years that we harbor reverberating wells of trauma in different parts of our body. My work centers on identifying where trauma may be hiding out in the body and releasing it by walking it through the Convergence Healing steps.

A traumatic experience can often throw someone into a pattern of lifelong pain. When trauma occurs we react on an unconscious "survive or die" level either by fighting, fleeing, freezing, or hiding. This reactive experience can live within us for decades. It does not matter how much the brain or conscious mind can identify and describe what happened. On a cellular level, our bodies identify only with the reaction they had. It does not matter if you have made peace with the event, forgiven your abuser, or healed all your physical wounds; the "survive or die" imprint remains.

For me, the "survive or die" moment came just a split second before I was slammed headfirst into that semitruck on that dark road so long ago. I remember having the thought that I ought to be able to keep myself from making contact, but then, the next thing I knew, I was being kicked out of heaven, only to return to earth with a broken body and a shattered spirit. It took me years of working on myself, years of querying my deepest self, to finally discover that I had the belief buried deep inside me that I should have somehow been able to stop the accident from happening. I also had deep deposits of shame about having survived—an experience my spirit processed as rejection. Lastly, great chunks of rage and anger got trapped within my broken bones, and it took me decades to be able to release these emotions.

The key to releasing all that traumatic residue? Love. The only true remedy for healing trauma is unconditional love. And lots and lots of it.

In the previous chapter, I wrote about how crucial trust is to healing, especially self-trust. If you are burdened with trauma, your ability to trust yourself has been doubly compromised. That's because we never know where, exactly, our traumatic wounds are and when they might be reactivated.

You know now, having read so much of my own story and having a sense of how Convergence Healing works, that I'm not an advocate of going back and reliving past trauma or in any way trying to provoke a traumatic response. What I do advocate is learning to read and identify those emotional responses in us that are prompted by our trauma. For me, this meant learning to understand that my hair-trigger temper was a traumatic reminder of my accident and that I might have to monitor my quick temper for the rest of my life. Actually acknowledging this, with deep love and kindness, brought me relief from my angry outbursts for the first time in my life. In other words, the energetic healing love of Convergence Healing was the first treatment I found that actually soothed and diluted my traumatic rage.

For me, trauma is a memory that has not yet found its place in one's history. Like that ghost that thinks it is still alive, untreated trauma does not know that its time or relevance has passed. We need to help that ghost find its way home so that it can finally be put to rest.

I remind clients while they are revisiting their trauma during our sessions that although they are experiencing the emotions of a traumatic event that occurred long ago, there is nothing currently in this moment that is harming them. A client's heart will pound, he or she may cry and reexperience a sense of terror—but it's not the actual, original terror. These are just memories of something from the past. They are ephemeral. They do not have the power to hurt us unless we allow them to. And I gently remind my clients of these truths so that they may release these sensations, these ghosts of past harms, and find true, lasting relief.

DARREN

Darren came to me after years of traditional talk therapy. Despite having spent thousands of dollars and hundreds of hours, he was still deeply haunted by his time in the military. He never saw hand-to-hand combat, but he was still deeply traumatized by what he witnessed while serving in the battle zone. Diagnosed with post-traumatic stress disorder (PTSD), Darren was incredibly frustrated that he still felt disconnected, was struggling with sleep issues, and was barely managing his anger.

He had been out of the military for close to a decade and he had a beautiful wife and an inquisitive young child. He worked as a commercial plumber and would find his anger flaring up regularly throughout the day. Coworkers would needle him and even do things to trigger his anger, and though he would joke about his temper, he secretly feared that one day he would lose control and do something violent.

Darren felt like he expended a tremendous amount of energy burying his anger with a "normal" temperament. And he did! I could feel how much pressure was built up inside him as he literally gave off the heat of buried anger as he sat in front of me.

We talked about how going numb was the only thing that felt safe to Darren, but how with Convergence Healing he could find safe and appropriate ways of releasing the pressure that had built up in his body, which was now manifesting as chronic stomachaches.

I asked Darren to gently hold his belly while we talked. He told me that while he was in Afghanistan, every time an ambulance horn would alert the compound that wounded were incoming, he would get such a terrible cramp in his abdomen that it would knock the breath right out of him. I asked him if he would breathe gently into that knotted sensation and to let me know if it had a color or texture or a smell. He said it was a gray haze with a burning smell, like burning tires and gasoline. This was the smell of war.

I asked him if he could see through this gray haze, and at first he said it was burning his eyes. I looked over and noticed that he had begun to weep.

"There is grief there, in this awful knot," I said.

"Yes. I hated the idea that my peers—men just like me—were coming back either maimed or, worse, dead. And here I was, just feet from them. Safe from harm."

"But were you safe from harm?" I asked.

"Physically, I suppose so," Darren replied. "Emotionally, no. I couldn't take all that carnage. It literally ate me up inside." With those words, he dropped his hands from his belly.

"How do you feel?" I asked.

"It's strange. All of a sudden, I feel lighter. Like the toxic ball in my gut has been removed."

We joked then, that maybe he had undergone a bit of psychic surgery, but there was truth in this. By talking so openly—and non-judgmentally—about how his wartime experiences had become lodged in his body, Darren was able to finally release them. He was able, right then and there, to put the ghost to rest.

The next day I received an e-mail from Darren saying that people at work had actually noticed there was something different about him. He also told me that the evening after our session he had played with his daughter for the first time in weeks and had also made love to his wife. He felt like he was finally "back in my own skin."

ANDREW

Andrew suffers from a painful case of Crohn's disease. This long-lasting inflammation of the gastrointestinal tract causes ulcers, abdominal pain, and diarrhea. Crohn's is serious, even life threatening, and a severe flare-up can prompt radical surgery. Not only is this condition painful, but it can cause great social anxiety, shame, and embarrassment.

Andrew was having a tough time of it. I asked him to tell me what his pain felt like. (Warning: this is a bit graphic.)

"It feels like I am literally being stabbed in my anus. There is such sharp pain. There. It makes me feel afraid and superemotional."

"What are you afraid of?" I asked.

"I am afraid of not being able to control my own bodily functions," he replied.

Crohn's was a source of almost constant trauma in Andrew's life, and he spent most of his time hiding out from his friends and family, being completely unwilling to risk experiencing an embarrassing episode in their presence. And while this coping mechanism gave him a sense of control over his disease, it only served to make him feel more ashamed of it.

I asked him what this pain and shame looked like.

Andrew saw the color red and had the faintest metallic taste in his mouth. I asked him if he felt like he had to hide from this sensation or if he could just "be" with it. He decided that he could tolerate it, and to his surprise, the pain he'd felt in his intestines all week subsided. He told me that, for the first time in days, he felt that he could relax. Now that he was a bit more at ease, I led him into the exercise Already Done.

My chi gong master originally shared the concept of "already done" with me. Our cells hold on to the messages we send them, and Andrew had been sending messages of pain and fear to his body all week long. I asked Andrew to take the phrase "already done" and to put that into the part of his body that was in pain. I asked him to visualize that phrase being repeated over and over again inside his body.

As Andrew was doing this, I guided him to feel the vibration of the words as he spoke them. We were both asking the part of him that was in pain to understand the meaning and feel the vibration of "already done" so that the pain would not be carried into Andrew's future. We were suggesting to his cells that the pain had passed. That they could relax and just be. That the pain was "already done."

Andrew has a deep appreciation for music, so I asked him to add some music to this mantra when he was doing this at home. He began to layer in drums and violins when he needed to use this phrase to quiet his pain, and so the vibrational healing pulse of this sound took on greater meaning for him and became a more effective tool of healing.

During our next session, we addressed the color of his pain. The red that Andrew saw around his pain gave way to a deep, tranquil turquoise blue—one of Andrew's favorite colors.

I asked Andrew to scan his body and, wherever he came upon an area that was hot, red, and inflamed, to wash it with turquoise-blue water, the water one would find on a perfect, sunny Caribbean day.

I asked him how this made him feel. The stabbing sensation that had tormented him for weeks gave way to a sensation of gentle pressure, almost like an internal hug.

"Holy crap, I don't have any more pain!" he blurted out.

We both laughed at his hilarious, inadvertent pun.

When I checked in with Andrew last, he had been using the "already done" mantra and the other Convergence Healing tools he'd gotten from his pain, and his life had blossomed in wonderful, unanticipated ways. He was embarking on a new romantic relationship—something he'd denied himself since being diagnosed with Crohn's several years ago—and was actively putting a great deal of work and effort into self-care. The results were impressive, especially in regard to his disease, which, he told me, had been in remission for several months.

Andrew still had Crohn's disease, but now he was pain-free. And loving it.

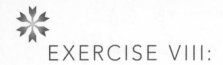

EXERCISE VIII:

A NEW SHADE OF HEALTH

Using color to facilitate healing has been in practice since at least 2000 BCE. Ancient texts tell of using color and light therapy to heal many maladies, and modern science uses color therapy to improve health in prisons, in hospitals, and, surprisingly, even in coal mines. Used as a treatment for a wide range of illnesses and diseases, these therapies, referred to as phototherapy and chromotherapy, are successful in treating mood disorders, depression, seasonal affective disorder (SAD), black lung disease, psoriasis, and even jaundice. According to Massachusetts Institute of Technology nutritionist Richard J. Wurtman, research has shown that individual colors influence respiration rates, blood pressure, biorhythms, and brain activity.

When we speak about our pain it is common to say things like "All I can see is red!" when we are angry or "Everything just went black" when we are overwhelmed and frustrated. Take a moment to tune in to the color of your pain. Be as specific as possible, as even a variation of a particular color can foster a deeper understanding of what you are contending with.

The color of my pain is _____.

Now take a moment to sit with that color. Acknowledge it and hold space for it. Notice where the color lives inside you and how it feels.

Once you have done this, invite a different color—one that you associate with health and feeling at ease—to take its place.

Let this new color fill up the space where the color of pain had been living.

The color of my wellness is _____.

You can build on this practice by incorporating your "wellness" color into your daily life. Look for ways to wear that color, paint a room that color, or get bedding in that shade. Even wearing a pair of socks in a wellness hue can be beneficial and enlivening. Have fun with it and know in confidence that every time you see that color you are sending a message of wellness into every cell of your being.

CHAPTER NINE

Embrace the Unknown

If you want to move to a higher level of life, you have to be willing to let go of some of your old ways of thinking and being and adopt new ones. The results will eventually speak for themselves.

—T. Harv Eker, *Secrets of the Millionaire Mind*

One of the unexpected benefits I gained from my own experience with Convergence Healing was how available I became to participating in life. My pain had made me self-absorbed. It had limited my ability to see beyond my own discomfort for so long that, when I did begin to feel better, I made very tentative steps back out into the world around me.

With a few solid years of my own healing under my belt, I found myself finally able to give back to my community. I'm now a proud homeowner in my Los Angeles neighborhood, having bought a fixer-upper bungalow and really turning the place around. When I felt more confident in my ability to take care of myself and my own property, I found myself wanting to care for a highway underpass not far from where I live, a place that's a magnet for troubled souls, drug dealings, and trash. It became really hard for me to have this dangerous eyesore in my life without at least trying to do something about it, so I galvanized my neighbors and enticed the entire junior high school down the street to work together to completely "renovate" the underpass. Together we painted four murals, worked with the city to put in new street signs and lighting, and planted trees. The Myra Avenue Mural Project was accomplished with donations and volunteers. I realized that my once-broken spirit was now soaring!

I was getting things done. I was connecting with people. I felt valuable and valid. And, slowly but surely, I became aware that I was learning to train my mind to stay focused on what is, not on what was or what might be. I started to want to be part of the solution, not mired in the problem, which is where pain had kept me for so long.

As I was able to recognize that I was making better decisions and developing a sense of trust, I began to experience a feeling of belonging that had eluded me for most of my life. I was becoming a truer, more authentic version of myself, and I was beginning to like it.

Part of what I had to do to deepen the experience of becoming myself was to allow myself to grieve. I had to grieve for all the time I had lost while I was invested in keeping the healthier, freer me pinned down. I had to acknowledge that, for a very long time, I had been addicted to mistrusting people, including myself. I had to let go of the "crutch" pain had become for me and bolster myself to stay firm, even when my steps were shaky or unsure. I had to release all the pent-up sorrow I'd accumulated by staying on the sidelines of life. And then I had to let all that grief go too.

This is when I stepped into the great unknown: the present moment, untainted by the past, not yet lost to the future. This is when I became fully aware of the here and now.

Staying in the present moment is the most challenging work I've ever done. At times it feels as though I'm wobbling along the thinnest wire, perched high above anything that looks or feels like safety. At other times I feel like I'm being embraced by a vast, limitless expanse of acceptance. Each day is like no other, and if I keep my expectations in check and really practice accepting "what is," I usually have a pretty fabulous day. My goal each day is to stay calm, centered, and at ease with myself, to protect myself as much as possible from injury (from others and myself).

I like this place. It's calm. It's balanced. But it's not always easy for me to stay the course. I'm just not a naturally calm and peaceful person. On the contrary! (I can't blame all my temperamental quirks on my accident.) But now, when I get tangled up in frustration or I feel my anger rising, I turn to the Convergence Healing tools that I know I can rely on.

Because these tools were given to me by my pain, they are a unique, very important part of who I am. They are gifts from the honest, unadorned, bedrock realities of Peter Bedard. They're not the "should" parts of me or the "what if" parts of me, and they're definitely not the "victim" parts of me; they're the hopeful, human, "I know I'm loved by this crazy, brilliant universe just as I am" parts of me. And when they're acknowledged and working in harmony, I feel whole and well.

I have learned by walking the Convergence Healing path that healing from our pain and becoming whole is a journey. It's a process that takes patience and a firm belief that the baby steps will lead to something significant.

The goal is to learn to accept yourself just as you are. In this very moment in time.

I still feel pain, of course. Convergence Healing hasn't turned me into a Vulcan (though that wouldn't be so bad, either). But now, instead of immediately becoming angry with my pain or resentful of it, I tune in to it to learn the lesson it wishes to impart. By learning to face my pain, I've not only grown up but I've gotten more resilient. I've become stronger and kinder. I've grown wiser but without all the arrogant self-righteousness that pain can bring with it. In short, I've become a much better man than I was before I let my pain change me.

So it goes without saying that, although change is usually served up with a big, heaping side of discomfort, that discomfort is worth it. For me, the more comfortable I became with change and the more willing I became to face the unknown, the more my fear yielded to a kindly curiosity about myself and the great big world I live in. There is a vast, wonderful world of experience beyond pain, and I want to explore it. I want to know it.

Releasing pain as the core of our identity means we go through a process of being broken apart so that we can be drawn back together with more harmony and health. Take, for instance, Humpty Dumpty: I'm certain he would be put back together again, and if done properly he would no longer be out of balance and so liable to fall and crack. When our pain is absent or neutralized, the mind, body, and spirit can fall into natural alignment, an alignment that reflects the true self. A self that faces the world without being blindfolded by pain.

Facing one's pain takes courage, and this is not a trait we value enough in ourselves. Turning to face trauma of any sort takes a strength of heart that reflects the best of humankind: the ability to stand tall when there are powerful forces, currents, or voices pushing against us. Tapping into this native courage is a groundbreaking experience for many people who have felt powerless when confronted with pain. Finding out that you have a certain level of grit—no matter what you're up against—taps into the unlimited resource of energetic love that will truly heal and transform you.

But shedding the identity we clung to when we were in pain isn't always easy. We have to be comfortable with the "in-between," the intangible, the undefined, the impermanent. This is when meditation, breathing, and self-hypnosis become such useful tools. When we step out of our identity as a "victim of pain," we have to hold steady while we simply . . . are.

I remember when my healing really began to take hold to the point that I'd catch myself doing something so normal—like driving to the market or walking my dog or laughing with a friend—and it would hit me: this is what life is like without the burden of pain. It was exhilarating and disorienting at once, and before my healing, this kind of moment would have triggered all kinds of anxiety within me because I was so used to tagging every waking moment by how it related to my pain. In fact, in the past, if I couldn't put an experience, thought, or feeling somewhere under that big black umbrella of pain, it would piss me off—because it made me feel like I didn't have control.

What a lie this was. What a lie it was that pain knew better than I did. What a lie it was that pain was more powerful than energetic love.

I'm still unlearning this, and I would say this is the greatest work of Convergence Healing: training the mind to resist being pulled back into the dark force field of the victim, the place where pain wants you to live.

This kind of training takes tenderness and absolute acceptance. Every little snipe, every morsel of judgment, keeps me from being truly pain-free. Taking care of myself, mind, body, and soul, is essential to this training. I simply have to wake up each morning and set the intention: I want to be free of pain.

HARRY

Harry is an executive in his early forties. He works for a new media company and was recently promoted. On the face of it, this was something to celebrate: he was given an impressive bump in pay and his visibility as a "face" of the brand was about to increase too.

But there was one problem. Harry's promotion meant that he'd be managing three times as many people as he had been, and this caused him great pain and concern.

I met him about six months into his new role as a managing director. He arrived at my office five minutes early and dressed in impeccable style. He looked fit and relaxed. Until he sat down.

"I have the strangest pain," he told me as he crossed his legs and wiggled his toes. My clients are asked to leave their shoes at the door. Harry did so but seemed uncomfortable with it.

I offered Harry a glass of water, then I asked him to describe his pain.

"Please don't laugh. I have the worst pain in my feet—but it only occurs when I'm off them. That's why I'm rubbing them now," he said.

I asked him to give me more detail about the pain, if he could. "It feels like there are dozens of very sharp needles that start to prick me from the inside out whenever my feet leave the ground.

It's absolutely at its worst in the middle of the night—at about three a.m.—when I most desperately need to sleep." He looked at his feet and frowned. "I've been to several top doctors—podiatrists, neurologists, even an endocrinologist to see if I had diabetes, but I'm the picture of good health. No one can explain it, and the only relief I've been offered is prescription sleep medication laced with pain medication. I live a pretty clean lifestyle and I need to stay superfocused at work, so that just wasn't an option.

"I've been white-knuckling it at work, operating on little sleep, and shuffling around on my feet all day, afraid that if I sit down, I'll lose it. But it's really taken a toll on my management skills. My coworkers feel like I'm trolling around to monitor them, and I'm grouchy and temperamental. They're all young kids, bright recent college grads, and I don't want to dump my middle-aged-man problems on them, so . . ."

"So you suffer in silence. Right?" I asked.

"Of course. I don't even know what I'm suffering from, so how can I talk about it?"

So many of us who are in pain have no idea why. There are millions and millions of people around the world hobbled by an undiagnosed or unacknowledged pain. A great example is the awful deep tissue pain experienced by those who suffer from chronic fatigue syndrome. Until recently, this complex virus was derided as the "yuppie flu" and those who suffered from it were considered lazy or neurotic. Now there is medical evidence to show that this kind of pain is not all in one's head.

I was certain that Harry's pain was all too real, and I wanted to help him find some relief.

I asked Harry if he would be comfortable lying down on the couch and putting his feet up. I assured him that I was not going to touch him; I just wanted to see if there was any activation of the pain he experienced when he was not standing.

So he lay down on the couch and we continued to chat.

Harry told me that he'd gone to an Ivy League school but that he'd felt like a bit of a faker there because he was admitted more for his prowess on the soccer field than for his great grades. He'd majored in business and landed with a great start-up in New York, where he met his wife. Or rather, his soon-to-be ex-wife. When they got together, she decided that the tech world wasn't for her, so she went back to school and studied literature. Then she got a teaching job at a small private school just outside the city. Not long after she started, the firm where they'd met went under and Harry lost all their money—money he'd reinvested in the company. He went for months without being able to find another job, and when he did, it was across the country.

The stress of his job loss and his dark moodiness while he was unemployed had taken a huge toll on his marriage. They agreed that he'd move out on his own and that they'd take this time as a "trial separation." That was just over a year ago. The painful pins and needles in his feet started shortly after he arrived, but became much worse when, six months into his "year off," his wife filed for divorce. Since then, he'd been in agony most nights.

"You miss her, don't you?" I asked.

"I do. Yes. But I feel like I've had to stay the course. You know?" he replied.

Boy, did I know. I knew how painful it was to feel like I had no choice but to lock myself into a role—even if that role didn't suit me at all.

I asked Harry if he'd been involved with anyone else, and he told me no—he just had not been interested. He still loved his wife.

Instead, he'd poured himself into his work, logging ridiculously long days, from seven in the morning to ten at night.

I asked him if he might be avoiding something important by filling his days—and nights—with only work.

"Yes," he said. "I'm avoiding coming home to an empty house and an empty bed."

There it was. Harry experienced intense pain in his feet whenever he went to bed, a bed he once shared with the woman he loved. This made perfect sense to me. Now I needed to find out if Harry could reach the same conclusion.

I asked Harry to close his eyes and led him into a light hypnotic state by doing a head-to-toe body scan. When we got down to his feet, I asked him if he was feeling any pain there.

"Yes. I feel those little knives jabbing at me," he said.

"Do they have a color?" I asked.

"Yes. They're red. Bright red," he answered.

"Is there any other quality about them you can share?" I asked.

"They've changed, actually. They're not like knives—they're more like hot coals that are stuck to the bottom of my feet," he said.

"This is a very good sign," I said. "It means the pain wants to leave your body. What else do you see or feel?"

"I want to run across them. I want to get to the cool water that is just beyond them," Harry said, his voice becoming emotional.

"Then let yourself do that. Let yourself step out of the burning coals and move onto cooler ground," I encouraged him.

When Harry had moved across the coals, I told him that the coals were now behind him, that he'd done the fire walk. And I asked him to repeat that it was "already done." Then I gently guided him out of the trance and back into the present moment.

When he sat up, he looked like a different man. He was calm, refreshed, and no longer clutching at his feet. I offered him another glass of cool water and he drank it down.

We chatted for another half hour, and Harry told me that he realized, having engaged in this brief hypnotic healing session, that he'd been punishing himself for his marriage failing ever since he'd lost his money and his job. Even though he was now a "success," he didn't know how to let himself off the hook.

"You just did," I said. "You just walked through the fire. It's already done."

I asked Harry to check in with me the next day. When he called, he told me that he'd slept well for the first time in a year and that he had experienced very little pain in his feet.

About six weeks later, my phone rang. It was Harry. He wanted me to know that he was doing well at work, and since he no longer felt compelled to stand all day, doing laps around the vast, open warehouse he worked in, his colleagues were able to relax and they were now working with much more ease. He was able to manage them by staying out of their way and, consequently, his division was thriving. He was also going to go on a date for the first time too: he'd called his ex-wife and told her how sorry he was. They spent the next few weeks reconnecting by phone, and he told me that at the end of the month he was going to meet her for a long weekend at a beach they both loved. He was hopeful. And grateful. And very glad to be living in the present moment.

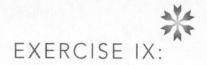

EXERCISE IX:

BALANCING IN THE NOW

Here's an exercise I offer to my clients. I think of it as a way to balance the scales between where we are (our perception of ourselves and our circumstances) and where we want to be. When we can honestly acknowledge both sides of this equation, we find a balancing point—right in the middle—that is this present moment. This point, which rests at perfect equilibrium between the way we perceive our current lives and what we wish our lives to be in the future, is the only moment that we really have. What's done is done. What hasn't happened yet, we cannot predict. But what we can do is be here, now, in this moment.

I find that when I do this written exercise myself, the disappointment I might feel in where I think I am is counterbalanced by the expectations I have about where I'd like to be. There is a balancing, a "canceling out," that occurs, and what I'm left with is just me, in this moment, free from judgment, despair, and expectation. Try this:

How do I feel physically?
Answer: (My knee aches.)

How do I want to feel physically?
Answer: (Strong and pain-free.)

How do I feel emotionally?

Answer: (I feel frustrated.)

How do I want to feel emotionally?
Answer: (Relaxed and comfortable.)

How do I feel in my spirit?	How do I want to feel in my spirit?
Answer: (Stuck, lost.)	Answer: (Loved and belonging.)

When we walk this path and lead with our heart—really speak our truth, with deep honesty—we point ourselves toward health and recovery. We orient ourselves away from pain and toward energetic love and healing.

CHAPTER TEN

Move into Action

Never a lip is curved with pain that can't be kissed into smiles again.

—Bret Harte

Your pain is the breaking of the shell that encloses your understanding.

—Kahlil Gibran

I decided to start this chapter with not one but two fabulous quotes that highlight the two most important components of Convergence Healing, which are (1) changing your thinking about your pain and about who you are, and (2) using this new point of view to propel you into healthy action.

When we take the time to witness our thinking and do the work of flushing out the antiquated, toxic, harmful thoughts that have kept us down in our pain, only then are we primed to take meaningful action and step with energetic love into our lives with greater ease, greater health—and more freedom from pain.

Convergence Healing is, above all, an action; it's about building an appetite for an authentic life and it's about oiling the wheels of our minds and hearts so that they can turn and propel us into a deeper state of awareness, a deeper state of love with life.

You've seen, with every client story I've shared, that it takes guts to be willing to name your pain, and I've been humbled and inspired by the hundreds of people who have come to me searching for a way to finally make peace with their pain. I've had the great honor and pleasure of watching these people, from all walks of life and from around the globe, take the first heroic step into their own healing by owning and naming their pain. Deniz is one of them.

DENIZ

"Would you please tell me where it hurts?" I asked the woman sitting before me. I was in Istanbul, Turkey, at a conference, and I was in front of a large audience, showing them how Convergence Healing works so that they could do it for themselves.

The woman, Deniz, tried to lift her right arm—with no success. Instead, she let out a yelp of pain. She was a young grandmother who told me, via an interpreter, that her right arm had been frozen and nearly useless for many months. She had come to the conference despairing that she would never be able to use her arm again and desperate to try anything, even if it meant, in her words, "learning a parlor trick." She sat before me, downcast, her arm locked rigid and straight at her side.

"My shoulder hurts. Here . . ." She tapped her right shoulder gently with her left hand. Her movements were slow and methodical, and her right arm hung still and immobile.

"What is your relationship with your shoulder?" I asked.

"It won't work. I hate it," she said.

"You hate it?" I asked. She was there, at the conference, because she had lost all tolerance for her pain. This was a good sign.

"I have things I need to do," she declared, waving her left hand and causing a ripple of nervous laughter in the audience. "It will not move. At all," she said. When she tried to move her right arm again, she grimaced in pain. She kept trying and her arm stayed stubbornly stiff, like it was not a part of her body.

"So it gets angry back at you. It rebels against you," I said. "It is important that we stay present with the parts of us that are hurting so that we can help them heal. Rather than making the pain an orphan, we can bring it closer to us. Deniz, would you be able to approach your arm, which is clearly injured, with more love and understanding?" I asked. As I spoke, the energy in the room began to change. Deniz nodded, then lifted her right hand ever so slightly.

"Did you see what she just did?" I asked the audience members, who were nodding enthusiastically.

"Very good." I turned to Deniz and said, "When you acknowledge your pain, without making it wrong or bad, it stops having so much control over you." She looked up at me, expectant and hopeful. "I am going to ask you to set an intention, just for today. Your arm, from your shoulder to the tip of your fingers, is going to move with grace and ease if you treat it with love and respect. Do you think you could do that?"

"Yes," she said, nodding.

"I am going to ask you to close your eyes and visualize the pain. Now I want you to visualize the pain moving out of your arm and into the world beyond your body." Deniz did as I asked and then let out a long-held breath. I could feel her relax beside me.

"What do you see?" I asked her. Often my clients will describe their pain as a color or a sensation (for example, as "hot" or "electric" or "frozen") or a sound (it "hums" or sounds like a "distant car alarm").

"It is a table with a pen on it," she said. As she spoke, she lifted her right arm significantly, her eyes still closed.

"It is a table with a pen on it," I repeated, intrigued. This was a rare occasion for me. In my experience, pain had never manifested as an inanimate object before.

"When I see this table and pen, I feel a burning ache in my right forearm," Deniz said.

"I would like you to gently cradle your right arm in your left and say out loud 'Just let it be.'" She did as I asked. "Just let it be," I stated again. I was asking her to let her arm physically know that it was loved.

She then continued. "This table is in a dark place." She was now describing the emotional facets of her pain. She was telling me—us—that she felt like she was in a dark place.

I asked her, "Can the darkness be okay?" Deniz assented, so I went on. "The table might have a name. Would you please ask its name?"

"Adige," she replied without hesitation.

"Hello, Adige," I offered. The audience before us was now spellbound. "Adige is part of you?" I asked.

"Yes," she answered in a whisper.

"She is not feeling very loved because you are frustrated with her," I said. "What if you actually showered Adige with love? What if you directed a beautiful golden light on her? What if you filled her with bright, healing energy? Lastly, I'd like you to ask Adige what she needs."

"She needs my attention" was her reply. "She needs me to listen to what she has to say."

"How can you do that physically?" I asked. "Physically, how can you let Adige know you love her?"

"By relaxing," responded Deniz, whose entire body seemed to soften as she spoke those words.

"Focus on sending relaxing thoughts and healing energy into your arm, which is where Adige has come from," I suggested.

The room was silent. While Deniz focused on relaxing her arm, I spoke to the assembled group: "What does it mean to really relax? What would that feel like? Is there a color you associate with deep, peaceful relaxation? Is there a temperature, an image, a sound, or a texture you experience when you are at peace? Most important, try to really embrace a physical knowing of what it means to be relaxed, and just let it be."

I watched Deniz relax and she began to gently swing her right arm, back and forth.

"How do you feel?" I gently inquired.

"I feel relaxed. Almost happy," she said, and a smile spread across her face.

"How does your arm feel now?" I asked.

"It feels young again!" she blurted out. The audience laughed.

"Are you ready to open your eyes?" I asked.

"Yes." She opened her eyes, and at the same time she lifted her once frozen arm even more.

"My arm is no longer separate from me," Deniz said.

"Good," I said. "Aside from your attention, what else might Adige [Deniz's pain] need from you?" I asked.

"She wants me to stop controlling others and she wants me to sit and read more, to allow myself to work less and learn more," Deniz replied.

She was spontaneously sharing what her soul needed when it was not paralyzed by pain.

"Everyone will have to take care of themselves if I relax," Deniz told me. Now the audience laughed freely, nodding in recognition of what she was saying.

"And if everyone took care of themselves, would that be okay?" I asked.

"Yes! I would love that," she replied.

I asked Deniz to stand up then and to see how high she could lift her arm. She was able to lift it straight over her head—without pain.

Deniz now has a "recipe" for dealing with her pain. She needs to catch herself when she becomes angry and judgmental with her exhaustion and her pain, and she needs to turn her love inward toward the parts of herself that she is frustrated with. In this case, it is her arm—an arm that she's clearly been overusing while caring for others.

"Thank you, thank you so much," she said in Turkish as she reached out to shake my hand vigorously with her previously immovable right hand.

WHAT DOESN'T KILL US
MAKES US STRONGER

Well, isn't that the truth! I know from my own years of living pinned down by pain that it wasn't until I decided I had to take action around my pain that I started to regain my strength and my desire to really live.

Coming into honest, direct contact with our pain breaks down all sorts of barriers we've built up around our authentic selves. Tearing down these defenses makes us so much more resilient. Pain gives us the chance to find out what we're truly made of; it allows our character to be forged in a necessary fire. Pain lets us discover our grit. And then—paradox of paradoxes—it softens us. Grit and kindness go hand in hand. Weakness, passivity, fear— these traits pair up with pain all too nicely. Once we understand that being victimized—allowing pain to weaken us—doesn't honor who we really are, we have no choice but to forge on to higher ground.

But it's a process, and a lifelong one at that. Releasing pain is like peeling an onion: there are layers and layers and more layers. But each release, each breakthrough, each gesture we make that supports our own health, restores us to ourselves.

Once I became serious about getting better, my pain began to recede, and with each day I became a little bit wiser and a lot more formidable. I was finally growing up and getting serious about my life.

I was becoming determined to be someone who contributes something positive to the world. If I had not been in that awful accident and died, sure, I may have gone on to have a career as a dancer, but I never, ever would have become a healer. I'm certain of that. Pain made me who I am—and that's something I'm proud of.

BANKING ON YOUR WELL-BEING

Every action you take—every gesture you make that is in service of your health—is like putting money in the Bank of You. It's really important to know this, because setbacks are normal and to be expected. If you're struggling, say, with the pain caused by binge eating, you must know, as you embark on your healing, that a slip or a binge is likely to happen. But every experience of healthy eating that you've consciously engaged in is now in your bank, fortifying you and protecting you as you continue on your journey of Convergence Healing.

Each day, invest in yourself by scanning yourself for pain. If you land on something that's causing you discomfort, greet that pain and then name it. When you've named it, ask it what it needs. Trust that the information it gives you will be honest and enlightening. Then take an action based on that information. I can guarantee that you will feel different. You will feel better. You will be, however, subtly transformed.

Every day is an opportunity for transformation. And every day is an opportunity to add more money to the bank of your well-being. This might mean drinking a glass of clean, fresh water upon waking. It might mean making sure you step away from your desk and take a walk in nature for at least twenty minutes. It might mean that you pick up the phone to call a friend and make amends. It can be any number of things—as long as it is an action that supports your feeling whole and healthy.

It is that simple. Convergence Healing is about becoming fully committed to your own health.

I love getting letters and notes from my clients telling me that their lives have changed for the better since they have begun following the practices of Convergence Healing. I get a "bump" of their energy each time I hear from one of them, and it furthers my own healing. Energetic love is what a meaningful life is all about and energetic love is all around us. It's our job to tap into it within ourselves and then share that joyful radiance with everyone we know. There is nothing like Convergence Healing to launch you out of your sense of "otherness" and into awareness of our oneness. But this approach is not all light and love. You will have to find your strength and be persistent. You will have to work at it. That's because when a body (or a spirit, or a mind) that has been at rest for too long begins to reawaken and move again, there is bound to be resistance. And resistance is a good thing.

RESISTANCE IS A SIGN THAT YOU ARE ON THE RIGHT PATH

Resistance to change is part of the human experience. We all are wired to take action and to rest. When we're out of balance (usually because of pain) we tend to have a traumatic reaction (either fighting, fleeing, freezing, or hiding). These four reactions are neatly divisible into two types: hyperaction and complete inaction. When you finally figure out how to pick yourself up mentally and then use this energy to propel yourself physically, it's inevitable that you'll bump up against the invisible universal force field of existential resistance. It's not unlike the shell of an egg or the chrysalis of a butterfly: everything that is being born anew has to push out against a protective layer in order to expand into the universe.

So don't let the natural resistance you will come up against stop you. Instead, get curious about that too. I have a lot of clients for whom the idea of going to a gym represents the physical manifestation of this resistance. For clients coming off physical injuries or disabilities, showing up at a gym feels as daunting as jumping out of an airplane at thirty-five thousand feet. But remember: baby steps. If you put your gym clothes on one day and only manage to check your mailbox—guess what? You've taken an action. The next day—or the next week—you may actually check in at the gym and visit the locker room. Guess what? You've taken another great step. We all need to be free to take a step forward, and take a step back—to allow ourselves to dance our way into change instead of kidding ourselves that it's a straight shot.

One step forward, two steps back. Then three steps forward, no steps back. In the end, moving past our pain and toward a brighter, healthier future is all that matters.

And remember, resistance is a good thing.

CONVERGE: BUILD YOUR
BEAUTIFUL TRIBE

One of the most crucial things I learned about my own healing was that I didn't have to go it alone. Not only did I not have to—I wasn't going to get better if I tried to do it alone. In fact,

I'd been stoic for so long that people around me started to think of me as being haughty and superior—when really what I felt inside was lost, scared, and lonely!

You get no points for being stoic and silent. Uh-uh. You have to name your pain and share this knowledge with those who love you or those who are there in support of you (like therapists, doctors, teachers, coaches, friends, and healers). It takes a village to heal, and it can take a village of support to live a happy life!

I'm not suggesting that you have to become the life of the party; it's about quality, not quantity, when it comes to the people we choose to have in our healthy lives. In my own experience, nothing compares with the ability to say a loving no to someone or something that we sense won't help us feel better. We've all had (or been) the friend who drains the energetic love out of a situation rather than contributing to it, and lying low around people, places, or things that compromise our sense of peace and serenity is healthy behavior.

But we humans are pack animals, and we're simply not meant to go it alone. I don't know anyone on this planet who doesn't experience a bump in their level of well-being when they're on the receiving end of a smile or a kind gesture. Conversely, I don't know anyone who doesn't feel better when they give a smile, help someone in need, or simply go the extra mile from time to time—simply because they know it will energize their love.

Communication. Collaboration. Community. They're all important components of Convergence Healing.

LEARN TO ASK FOR HELP

Learning to ask for help is an incredibly empowering experience. It took me a long, long time to feel important enough and to get my ego out of the way before being able to humbly ask for help. When I did, *everything* in my life changed for the better. Asking for help in a nonmanipulative, genuine way is like putting a neon sign over your head that says "A Real Human Person Lives Here!"

When you reach out for another's hand, you invite tenderness to surround you. This is something that I feel, in spades, when I'm doing a session with a client. There is always a lot of vulnerability in the room, all the way around. I'm always nervous about whether I'll be able to "help" someone; I know that I can help them, but I worry that they will not be able to take in and process my message.

Sometimes clients come to me with such traumatic experiences that I have to wonder whether I can help them. I calm and center myself by reminding myself that I'm simply facilitating another person's ability to heal oneself. Then I trust the process, let go of my worry, and dive in. It has never failed me or a client. When that vulnerability is met with true curiosity and true compassion, there's a rush of tenderness that envelops the session, a sense of such gentle care that I am, frankly, at a loss to find the words to describe it without sounding too corny.

So learn to ask for help. And thank those who show up for you with open, authentic hearts, minds, and arms. When this happens, you are in the presence of the highest form of energetic love, and every fiber of your being will benefit from it.

BE LOVING

Be loving with yourself. Be loving with your pain. Be loving with others. A sense of caring is crucial to healing. Study after study shows that those who feel loved and who love recover the most rapidly from all types of illnesses and injuries. We've all heard tales of miraculous spontaneous recovery when someone who is ill or dying is being prayed for by strangers across the globe. It happens. It's real. Love really does heal. So be loving. Be love.

COMMIT TO BEING YOURSELF

Again, it's another cliché. But guess what? There is only one you, and, more important, you cannot be anyone other than you. Isn't that a relief? It's also pretty fantastic news. When we accept our uniqueness, we stop seeing our flaws and instead we begin to see our potential.

Ask yourself the juiciest questions:

> Who are you?
> What do you love?
> How do you want to spend your days?

And then let the answers blossom and flower in your heart until you're bursting with joyful, energetic love.

And if you're in pain? Now's your chance to explore who you are in pain, and when you decide you want to go deeper and find out who you are beneath the pain, then the real adventure begins.

Remember: you are not your pain. You are the glorious human being beneath the pain. Make a commitment to get to know this extraordinary person.

A Prayer to Be Pain-Free

Dear Pain,

Thank you for teaching me to love more deeply. Thank you for showing me how to heal and live my fullest life. Thank you for reminding me that I am powerful. Thank you for revealing my strengths, for showing me my weaknesses, and for embracing me with energetic love. Thank you for the healing. And so it is . . .

With love and gratitude.
Amen.

ACKNOWLEDGMENTS

I am grateful! I am grateful for the accident that killed me. I am grateful for the depression and anxiety that taught me how to love. I am grateful for the pain that slowed me down and required me to be present and breathe. I am grateful for my parents and their courage and love. I am grateful for my friends and family (for me, they are the same)—Dawn, McKerrin, George, Justino, Johnny, Greg, Aunty D, Mary Helen, Patricia, Pepe. I am grateful for the thousands of clients I have worked with in my practice and met through ConvergenceHealing.com for sharing their lives and teaching me ever-deeper experiences of love. I am grateful for Brian, Emily, Nancy, Thomas, and Zhena, and everyone at Enliven, Atria, and Simon & Schuster for helping me make my dreams come true. I am grateful for the community that embraces the work I do and for the amazing souls who help me create wellness wherever I go. And I am grateful for you! Thanks for letting me be of service.

—Peter Bedard
XO

ACKNOWLEDGMENTS

A book of this nature involves the guidance, inspiration, and knowledge of many others; to attempt to name all to whom I feel indebted would be another chapter unto itself. I do extend love and thankfulness to my parents; my brother and his family; my close, funny circle of friends; the Center for Spiritual Living Los Angeles; Steve Lapuk; and Franklin, whose love, laughter, strength, and grace have supported me since that night we met in Silver Lake. I am also grateful to Peter for his unwavering friendship, honesty, loyalty, and, most of all, my ongoing Convergence Healing.

—*Brian Sheffield Hunt*

CONVERGENCE HEALING
RESOURCE LIST

BOOKS TO READ TO HELP YOUR HEALING

The Alchemist by Paulo Coelho
This book is a mystical masterpiece that delivers on its message to follow our dreams.

Back in Control by David Hanscom, MD
The book by this talented surgeon is an inspiration for anyone struggling with back pain.

The Edinburgh and Dore Lectures on Mental Science
by Thomas Troward
This book, a milestone in metaphysical reasoning, is a cornerstone of both the New Thought and Science of Mind movements, as well as the Centers for Spiritual Living.

The Essential Rumi by Rumi
A book of poems by one of my favorites. His writings, including this quote "The cure for the pain is in the pain," continue to inspire me today.

The Four Agreements by don Miguel Ruiz

This book's essential steps toward a path to personal freedom are rooted in traditional Toltec wisdom.

Guided Imagery for Self-Healing by Martin L. Rossman, MD, www.thehealingmind.org

A book by Dr. Rossman, who, along with Dr. Dressler at the UCLA Pain Clinic, was a profound inspiration for my work.

Hyperbole and a Half by Allie Brosh

This book is as funny as it is smart, taking an inventive peek at how childhood molds our future.

Lessons of Truth by Rev. Marian G. Moon, www.csl-la.org

A book of short essays that will expand your ideas about the unmatched powers of the mind.

On Abundance and Right Livelihood by Neal Donald Walsch

This book has amazing inspiration to share and wisdom to spare.

The Power of Decision by Raymond Charles Barker

A book considered to be a classic must-read for any reader hoping for a better life by making better decisions.

The Power of Now by Eckhart Tolle

This book has a bold, simple message: living in the now is the truest path to happiness and enlightenment.

The Science of Mind by Ernest Holmes

This book outlines the foundational viewpoints of the modern New Thought movement. Born in 1887 on a small farm in Maine, Dr. Holmes spent his early years outdoors asking himself the ubiquitous questions "What is God?" "Who am I?" and "Why am I here?"

Secrets of the Millionaire Mind by Dr. T. Harv Eker

A book of true inspiration that is similar in context to Convergence Healing but focuses on financial healing and abundance.

The Self-Aware Universe by Amit Goswami, PhD

This book (one of my favorites!) is amazing. Dr. Goswami set out to become a scientist to disprove the existence of God but instead became a physicist theologian.

The Seven Spiritual Laws of Success by Deepak Chopra

A book detailing seven laws found in nature that can be used to create spiritual success.

Swamplands of the Soul by James Hollis

A book, dry but inspiring, on working through grief, depression, betrayal, etc.

Tuesdays with Morrie by Mitch Albom

This book is a touching account of a dying man relating his ideas of love, shunning the zeitgeist in favor of more nurturing values.

The Velvet Rage by Alan Downs, PhD

A book that focuses on healing lesbian and gay issues, yet anyone struggling with excessive shame will greatly benefit from this read.

The Worst Is Over: What to Say When Every Moment Counts—Verbal First Aid to Calm, Relieve Pain, Promote Healing, and Save Lives by Judith Acosta and Judith Simon Prager

A book by one of my mentors, Mrs. Prager, that was an inspiration in my early healing work.

You Are Enough by Dr. David J. Walker

A book written by a man who taught his life-changing philosophy of breaking out of restrictive patterns for over thirty groundbreaking years.

You Can Heal Your Life by Louise Hay

A book by the famed author who, upon being diagnosed with cancer, considered alternatives to surgery and drugs, instead developing an intensive program of affirmations, visualizations, nutritional cleansing, and psychotherapy that left her completely healed within six months.

TO LEARN MORE ABOUT HYPNOTISM

Hypnosis Motivation Institute—www.hypnosis.edu

A fantastic school, my alma mater, and a perfect resource for learning more about hypnosis.

Hypnothoughts—www.hypnothoughts.com

This international community of hypnotherapists hosts an annual conference in Las Vegas, Nevada.

National Guild of Hypnotists—www.ngh.net

The guild is a great way to locate vetted hypnotists in your area.

National Institutes of Health—www.nih.gov, www.ncbi.nlm.nih.gov/pmc/articles/PMC2752362

This national association offers insightful studies on hypnosis, how it works, and how it is being used to help those in pain to heal.

EVEN MORE WAYS TO HELP HEAL YOUR PAIN

Al-Anon Family Groups—www.al-anon.org

This international organization offers supportive literature and group meetings for the family and friends of those recovering from the effects of someone else's addiction.

Dr. Roger C. Barnes—www.drrogerbarnes.com

This doctor worked with me to eliminate an allergy to chlorine. His work is very effective.

Rickie Byars-Beckwith, and the Sound of Agape— www.soundofagape.com

One of my favorite songs that always lifts my heart is Rickie's rendition of "I Release and Let Go."

Centers for Spiritual Living—www.csl.org

A spiritual movement begun by Dr. Ernest Holmes (1887–1960) inspired this organization of nearly 400 spiritual communities around the globe that teach powerful principles for personal growth and global transformation, honoring all spiritual paths.

Create Your Health—www.createyourhealth.com

My website with over 60 videos of me experimenting with different healing therapies, as well as a healing tea store, Create Your Health Teas.

**The Holistic Chamber of Commerce—
www.holisticchamberofcommerce.com**

A fantastic online resource for finding a holistic or alternative therapist.

**Parents, Families and Friends of Lesbians and Gays
(PFLAG)—www.community.pflag.org**

An organization supporting lesbian, gay, bisexual, transgender, and queer (LGBTQ) with families, friends, and allies, PFLAG is committed to advancing equality and full societal affirmation of LGBTQ people through support meetings, education, and advocacy.

Prolotherapy—www.prolotherapyinstitute.com

This therapy guided me to discipline my mind through meditation, to sit and be still with the pain in my knee, and to walk through the pain almost daily. It also guided me to Dr. Marc Darrow, who helped me regenerate cartilage in my knee.

Qigong—www.chilel.com

Qigong is an ancient Chinese healing art—a practice I continue to use to this day. "Qi," or "chi," means "life energy," and "gong" means "daily effort." Starting with Dr. Frank Qigong and Dr. Luke Chan, I was able to heal my chronic sinus infections.

University of Philosophical Research—www.uprs.edu

The university where I studied to receive my MA in Consciousness Studies was founded in the early twentieth century. They have an incredible resource library.

CONVERGENCE HEALING
CHEAT SHEET

Always remember . . . love your gift of pain.

The key to Convergence Healing is saturating all parts of you with love on every level. This isn't just the thought of love but the actual experience. Know the color, sound, look, etc., of this love! Use this love to develop a healthy relationship with the part of you that is in pain and let it lead the way through your garden of healing.

Pain is not your enemy.

Pain in itself does not have to be a burden that keeps you imprisoned. Taking personal responsibility and identifying pain for what it actually is, the intimate private messenger that holds the answers to your healing, will free you from your suffering.

Name your pain and make it your best friend.

Communicate with your pain. Give it a name and, like a best friend that has come to you for help, love it so that you can work together to create a plan for your healing.

Step out of the fog.

No denying your pain or letting it run the show. Commit to being present in your better, ever-evolving state of awareness and step into your place of power where you call the shots.

Develop a convergent mind.

Control is a waste of time. Learn to discipline your thoughts and practice living in the governance of an open mind and heart.

Integrate your trauma.

Already done. Teach the experience of trauma that it is already done. Let it find its way back into your personal history. Understand that trauma is a memory, a ghost who does not know it has passed.

Love inside out.

Release shame by practicing loving yourself exactly as you are—good, bad, ugly—and nurture gratitude.

Develop trust in yourself.

Develop a recipe for healing your pain by asking the part of you that is in pain three basic questions. Remember: "The cure for the pain is in the pain."

1. What do I need to do to heal this pain on a mind level of being?

2. What do I need to do to heal this pain on a body level of being?

3. What do I need to do to heal this pain on a spirit level of being?

Move in action every day.

Embrace the freedom and wellness that comes from incorporating the Convergence Healing process into your daily life. Remember: you are not your pain. You are the glorious human being beneath the pain. Make a commitment to get to know this wonderful person and share the energetic love that is your healing.

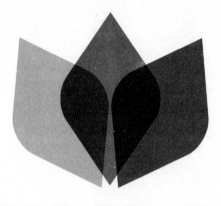

ENLIVEN™

About Our Books: We are the world's first holistic publisher for mission-driven authors. We curate, create, collaborate on, and commission sophisticated, fresh titles and voices to enhance your spiritual development, success, and wellness pursuits.

About Our Vision: Our authors are the voice of empowerment, creativity, and spirituality in the twenty-first century. You, our readers, are brilliant seekers of adventure, unexpected stories, and tools to transform yourselves and your world. Together, we are change-makers on a mission to increase literacy, uplift humanity, ignite genius, and create reasons to gather around books. We think of ourselves as instigators of soulful exchange.

Welcome to the wondrous world of Enliven Books, a new imprint from Zhena Muzyka, author of *Life by the Cup: Inspiration for a Purpose-Filled Life*, and Atria, an imprint of Simon & Schuster, Inc.

To explore our list of books and learn about fresh new voices in the realm of Mind-Body-Spirit, please visit us at

EnlivenBooks.com | ⑤/EnlivenBooks

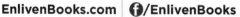